SOAP
for
Cardiology

Look for other books in this series!

SOAP for Emergency Medicine

SOAP for Family Medicine

SOAP for Internal Medicine

SOAP for Neurology

SOAP for Obstetrics and Gynecology

SOAP for Orthopedics

SOAP for Pediatrics

SOAP for Urology

SOAP
for
Cardiology

Eric H. Awtry, MD, FACC
Director of Education, Cardiology
Boston University Medical Center
Assistant Professor of Medicine
Boston University School of Medicine
Boston, Massachusetts

M. Faisal Khan, MD, MRCP
Cardiology Research Fellow
Harvard Medical School & Department of Clinical Biometrics
Brigham and Women's Hospital
Boston, Massachusetts

Jeremy B. Sokolove, MD
Chief Medical Resident
Boston University Medical Center
Boston, Massachusetts

Series Editor
Peter S. Uzelac, MD, FACOG
Assistant Professor
Department of Obstetrics and Gynecology
University of Southern California Keck School of Medicine
Los Angeles, California

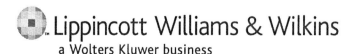
Lippincott Williams & Wilkins
a Wolters Kluwer business
Philadelphia · Baltimore · New York · London
Buenos Aires · Hong Kong · Sydney · Tokyo

Acquisitions Editor: Donna Balado
Managing Editor: Kathleen Scogna
Marketing Manager: Jennifer Kuklinski
Production Editor: Jennifer Glazer
Designer: Meral Dabcovich
Compositor: International Typesetting and Composition in India
Printer: Courier—Westford

Printed in the United States of America

Library of Congress Cataloging-in-Publication Data

Awtry, Eric.
  SOAP for cardiology / Eric H. Awtry, M. Faisal Khan, and Jeremy B. Sokolove.
      p. ; cm. — (SOAP series)
  Includes bibliographical references and index.
    ISBN-13: 978-1-4051-0472-2 (alk. paper)
    ISBN-10: 1-4051-0472-4 (alk. paper)
   1. Cardiology—Handbooks, manuals, etc. 2. Cardiovascular system—Diseases—Handbooks, manuals, etc. I. Khan, M. Faisal.
  II. Sokolove, Jeremy B. III. Title. IV. Series.
   [DNLM: 1. Cardiac Diseases—Handbooks. WG 39 A967s 2007]
RC669.15.A96 2007
616.1′2—dc22

                                                                                          2005037295

06 07 08 09 10
1 2 3 4 5 6 7 8 9 10

Contents

Reviewers ix
To the Reader xi
Abbreviations xii
Normal Laboratory Values xv

1. Chest Pain 2
2. Dyspnea 4
3. Palpitations 6
4. Syncope 8
5. Sudden Cardiac Death 10
6. Prinzmetal's (Variant) Angina 12
7. Stable Angina 14
8. Unstable Angina and Non–ST Segment Elevation
   Myocardial Infarction 16
9. ST Elevation Myocardial Infarction 18
10. Cardiac Stress Testing 20
11. Systolic Heart Failure 22
12. Diastolic Heart Failure 24
13. Right Heart Failure 26
14. Hypertrophic Cardiomyopathy 28
15. Dilated Cardiomyopathy 30
16. Myocarditis 32
17. Cardiogenic Shock 34
18. Acute Pericarditis 36
19. Pericardial Effusion 38
20. Pericardial Tamponade 40
21. Constrictive Pericarditis 42
22. Dressler's Syndrome 44
23. Mitral Stenosis 46
24. Aortic Stenosis 48
25. Mitral Regurgitation 50
26. Aortic Insufficiency 52
27. Tricuspid Regurgitation 54
28. Endocarditis 56
29. Ventricular Septal Defect 58
30. Atrial Septal Defect 60
31. Bicuspid Aortic Valve 62
32. Pulmonary Stenosis 64
33. Marfan Syndrome 66
34. Adult Congenital Heart Disease 68
35. First-Degree Atrioventricular Heart Block 70
36. Second-Degree Atrioventricular Heart Block 72
37. Third-Degree Atrioventricular Heart Block/Complete Heart Block 74
38. Wide Complex Tachycardia 76
39. Atrial Fibrillation 78
40. Atrial Flutter 80
41. Sick Sinus Syndrome 82

42. Wolff-Parkinson-White Syndrome 84
43. Atrioventricular Nodal Reentrant Tachycardia 86
44. Ventricular Tachycardia 88
45. Essential Hypertension 90
46. Secondary Hypertension 92
47. Hypertensive Emergency 94
48. Aortic Dissection 96
49. Peripheral Arterial Disease 98
50. Aortic Coarctation 100
51. Asymptomatic Carotid Bruit 102
52. Transient Ischemic Attack 104
53. Ischemic Cerebrovascular Accident 106
54. Pulmonary Hypertension 108
55. Thromboangiitis Obliterans (Buerger's Disease) 110
56. Atrial Myxoma 112
57. Cardiac Contusion 114
58. Hyperlipidemia 116
59. Elevated C-Reactive Protein 118
60. Hyperhomocystinemia 120
61. Coronary Calcium Score 122
62. Left Ventricular Hypertrophy 124

Index 127

Reviewers

Stephen Liu
Class of 2005
University of Maryland College of Medicine
Baltimore, Maryland

Cecelia Powless
Class of 2005
Southern Illinois University School of Medicine
Springfield, Illinois

Melanie Stickrath
Class of 2005
Medical College of Ohio
Toledo, Ohio

To the Reader

Like most medical students, I started my ward experience head-down and running, eager to finally make contact with real patients. What I found was a confusing world, completely different from anything I had known during the first 2 years of medical school. New language, foreign abbreviations, and residents too busy to set my bearings straight: Where would I begin?

Pocket textbooks, offering medical knowledge in a convenient and portable package, seemed to be the logical solution. Unfortunately, I found myself spending valuable time sifting through large amounts of text, often not finding the answer to my question, and in the process, missing out on teaching points during rounds!

I designed the SOAP series to provide medical students and house staff with pocket manuals that truly serve their intended purpose: quick accessibility to the most practical clinical information in a user-friendly format. At the inception of this project, I envisioned all of the benefits the SOAP format would bring to the reader:

• Learning through this model reinforces a thought process that is already familiar to students and residents, facilitating easier long-term retention.

• SOAP promotes good communication between physicians and facilitates the teaching/learning process.

• SOAP puts the emphasis back on the patient's clinical problem and not the diagnosis.

• In the age of managed care, SOAP meets the challenge of providing efficiency while maintaining quality.

• As sound medical-legal practice gains attention in physician training, SOAP emphasizes adherence to a documentation style that leaves little room for potential misinterpretation.

Rather than attempting to summarize the contents of a thousand-page textbook into a miniature form, the SOAP series focuses exclusively on guidance through patient encounters. In a typical use, "finding out where to start" or "refreshing your memory" with SOAP books should be possible in less than a minute. Subjects are always confined to two pages and the most important points have been highlighted. Topics have been limited to those problems you will most commonly encounter repeatedly during your training and contents are grouped according to the hospital or clinic setting. Facts and figures that are not particularly helpful to surviving life on the wards, such as demographics, pathophysiology and busy tables and graphs have purposely been omitted (such details are much better studied in a quiet environment using large and comprehensive texts).

Congratulations on your achievements thus far and I wish you a highly successful medical career!

Peter S. Uzelac, MD, FACOG

Abbreviations

A_2:	aortic component of the second heart sound
ABI:	ankle-brachial index
ACS:	acute coronary syndrome
ACE(I):	angiotensin-converting enzyme (inhibitor)
AFL:	atrial flutter
AF:	atrial fibrillation
AI:	aortic insufficiency
AIVR:	accelerated idioventricular rhythm
AMI:	acute myocardial infarction
ANA:	antinuclear antibody
APC:	atrial premature complex
ARB:	angiotensin receptor blocker
AS:	aortic stenosis
ASD:	atrial septal defect
AV:	aortic valve
AVB:	atrioventricular block
AV node:	atrioventricular node
AVNRT:	atrioventricular nodal reentrant tachycardia
AVRT:	atrioventricular reentrant tachycardia
BBB:	bundle branch block
BID:	twice daily
BNP:	brain natriuretic peptide
BP:	blood pressure
BPM:	beats per minute
BUN:	blood urea nitrogen
CAD:	coronary artery disease
CABG:	coronary artery bypass graft
CCS:	coronary calcium score
CHB:	complete heart block
CHD:	congenital heart disease
CHF:	congestive heart failure
CK:	creatinine kinase
CMP:	cardiomyopathy
COPD:	chronic obstructive pulmonary disease
CPAP:	continuous positive airway pressure
CRP:	C-reactive protein
CSM:	carotid sinus massage
CT:	computed tomography
CV:	cardioversion
CVA:	cerebrovascular accident
DCM:	dilated cardiomyopathy
DHF:	diastolic heart failure
DM:	diabetes mellitus
dP/dT:	change in pressure/change in time
DVT:	deep venous thrombosis
EBCT:	electron beam CT
ECG:	electrocardiogram

EF:	ejection fraction
EP(S):	electrophysiological (study)
ESR:	erythrocyte sedimentation rate
GERD:	gastroesophageal reflux disease
HB:	heart block
HCM:	hypertrophic cardiomyopathy
HDL:	high-density lipoprotein
HF:	heart failure
HIV:	human immunodeficiency virus
HOCM:	hypertrophic obstructive cardiomyopathy
HR:	heart rate
HTN:	hypertension
ICD:	implantable cardioverter-defibrillator
ICU:	intensive care unit
IE:	infectious endocarditis
INR:	international normalized ratio
JVP:	jugular venous pressure (or pulse)
LA:	left atrium
LBBB:	left bundle branch block
LDL:	low-density lipoprotein
LFT:	liver function test
LV:	left ventricle
LVH:	left ventricular hypertrophy
LVEF:	left ventricular ejection fraction
MAO(I):	monoamine oxidase (inhibitor)
MAP:	mean arterial pressure
MAT:	multifocal atrial tachycardia
MEN:	multiple endocrine neoplasia
MET:	metabolic equivalent
MI:	myocardial infarction
MR:	mitral regurgitation
MRA:	magnetic resonance angiography
MRI:	magnetic resonance imaging
MRSA:	methicillin-resistant *Staphylococcus aureus*
MS:	mitral stenosis
MV:	mitral valve
MVP:	mitral valve prolapse
NCEP:	National Cholesterol Education Program
NSAID:	nonsteroidal anti-inflammatory drugs
NSTE:	non-ST elevation (MI)
NSVT:	nonsustained ventricular tachycardia
NTG:	nitroglycerin
NYHA:	New York Heart Association
P_2:	pulmonic component of the second heart sound
PA:	pulmonary artery
PAC:	premature atrial complex
PAD:	peripheral arterial disease
PAT:	paroxysmal atrial tachycardia
PDA:	patent ductus arteriosus
PE:	pulmonary embolism

PFO:	patent foramen ovale
PHTN:	pulmonary hypertension
PMI:	point of maximal impulse
PND:	paroxysmal nocturnal dyspnea
PS:	pulmonic stenosis
PUD:	peptic ulcer disease
PV:	pulmonary valve
PVC:	premature ventricular complex
PVR:	pulse volume recording, pulmonary vascular resistance
QD:	once daily
Qp:	pulmonary blood flow
Qs:	systemic blood flow
RBBB:	right bundle branch block
RA:	right atrium
RF:	rheumatic fever, or radio frequency (ablation)
RV:	right ventricle
RVH:	right ventricular hypertrophy
S_1:	first heart sound
S_2:	second heart sound
S_3:	third heart sound
S_4:	fourth heart sound
SA:	sinoatrial
SBP:	systolic blood pressure
SCD:	sudden cardiac death
SLE:	systemic lupus erythematosus
SSS:	sick sinus syndrome
STE:	ST elevation (MI)
SVT:	supraventricular tachycardia
TAO:	thromboangiitis obliterans
TB:	tuberculosis
TC:	total cholesterol
TEE:	transesophageal echocardiography
TFT:	thyroid function test
TG:	triglyceride
TIA:	transient ischemic attack
TID:	three times daily
TPA:	tissue plasminogen activator
TR:	tricuspid regurgitation
TSH:	thyroid-stimulating hormone
TTE:	transthoracic echocardiography
TV:	tricuspid valve
UA:	unstable angina
VF:	ventricular fibrillation
VMA:	vanillylmandelic acid
VPC:	ventricular premature complex
VQ:	ventilation:perfusion (scan)
VSD:	ventricular septal defect
VT:	ventricular tachycardia
WCT:	wide complex tachycardia
WPW:	Wolff-Parkinson-White

Normal Laboratory Values

Blood, Plasma, Serum

Aminotransferase, alanine (ALT, SGPT)	0–35 U/L
Aminotransferase, aspartate (AST, SGOT)	0–35 U/L
Ammonia, plasma	40–80 µg/dL
Amylase, serum	0–130 U/L
Antistreptolysin 0 titer	Less than 150 units
Bicarbonate, serum	23–28 meq/L
Bilirubin, serum	
Total	0.3–1.2 mg/dL
Direct	0–0.3 mg/dL
Blood gases, arterial (room air)	
Po_2	80–100 mm Hg
Pco_2	35–45 mm Hg
pH	7.38–7.44
Calcium, serum	9–10.5 mg/dL
Carbon dioxide content, serum	23–28 meq/L
Chloride, serum	98–106 meq/L
Cholesterol, total, plasma	150–199 mg/dL (desirable)
Cholesterol, low-density lipoprotein (LDL), plasma	≤130 mg/dL (desirable)
Cholesterol, high-density lipoprotein (HDL), plasma	≥40 mg/dL (desirable)
Complement, serum	
C3	55–120 mg/dL
Total	37–55 U/mL
Copper, serum	70–155 µg/dL
Creatine kinase, serum	30–170 U/L
Creatinine, serum	0.7–1.3 mg/dL
Ethanol, blood	<50 mg/dL
Fibrinogen, plasma	150–350 mg/dL
Folate, red cell	160–855 ng/mL
Folate, serum	2.5–20 ng/mL
Glucose, plasma	
Fasting	70–105 mg/dL
2 hours postprandial	<140 mg/dL
Iron, serum	60–160 µg/dL
Iron binding capacity, serum	250–460 µg/dL
Lactate dehydrogenase, serum	60–100 U/L
Lactic acid, venous blood	6–16 mg/dL
Lead, blood	<40 µg/dL
Lipase, serum	<95 U/L

Magnesium, serum	1.5–2.4 mg/dL
Manganese, serum	0.3–0.9 ng/mL
Methylmalonic acid, serum	150–370 nmol/L
Osmolality plasma	275–295 mosm/kg H_2O
Phosphatase, acid, serum	0.5–5.5 U/L
Phosphatase, alkaline, serum	36–92 U/L
Phosphorus, inorganic, serum	3–4.5 mg/dL
Potassium, serum	3.5–5 meq/L
Protein, serum	
Total	6.0–7.8 g/dL
Albumin	3.5–5.5 g/dL
Globulins	2.5–3.5 g/dL
Alpha$_1$	0.2–0.4 g/dL
Alpha$_2$	0.5–0.9 g/dL
Beta	0.6–1.1 g/dL
Gamma	0.7–1.7 g/dL
Rheumatoid factor	<40 U/mL
Sodium, serum	136–145 meq/L
Triglycerides	<250 mg/dL (desirable)
Urea nitrogen, serum	8–20 mg/dL
Uric acid, serum	2.5–8 mg/dL
Vitamin B_{12}, serum	200–800 pg/mL

Cerebrospinal Fluid

Cell count	0–5 cells/µL
Glucose	40–80 mg/dL
(less than 40% of simultaneous plasma concentration is abnormal)	
Protein	15–60 mg/dL
Pressure (opening)	70–200 cm H_2O

Endocrine

Adrenocorticotropin (ACTH)	9–52 pg/mL
Aldosterone, serum	
Supine	2–5 ng/dL
Standing	7–20 ng/dL
Aldosterone, urine	5–19 µg/24 h
Cortisol	
Serum 8 am	8–20 µg/dL
5 pm	3–13 µg/dL
1 h after cosyntropin	>18 µg/dL
usually ≥8 µg/dL above baseline	
overnight suppression test	<5 µg/dL

Urine free cortisol	<90 µg/24 h
Estradiol, serum	
Male	10–30 pg/mL
Female	
Cycle day 1–10	50–100 pmol/L
Cycle day 11–20	50–200 pmol/L
Cycle day 21–30	70–150 pmol/L
Estriol, urine	>12 mg/24 h
Follicle-stimulating hormone, serum	
Male (adult)	5–15 mU/mL
Female	
Follicular or luteal phase	5–20 mU/mL
Midcycle peak	30–50 mU/mL
Postmenopausal	>35 mU/mL
Insulin, serum (fasting)	5–20 mU/L
17-ketosteroids, urine	
Male	8–22 mg/24 h
Female	Up to 15 µg/24 h
Luteinizing hormone, serum	
Male	3–15 mU/mL (3–15 U/L)
Female	
Follicular or luteal phase	5–22 mU/mL
Midcycle peak	30–250 mU/mL
Postmenopausal	>30 mU/mL
Parathyroid hormone, serum	10–65 pg/mL
Progesterone	
Luteal	3–30 ng/mL
Follicular	<1 ng/mL
Prolactin, serum	
Male	<15 ng/mL
Female	<20 ng/mL
Testosterone, serum	
Adult male	300–1200 ng/dL
Female	20–75 ng/dL
Thyroid function tests (normal ranges vary)	
Thyroid iodine (^{131}I) uptake	10% to 30% of administered dose at 24 h
Thyroid-stimulating hormone (TSH)	0.5–5.0 µU/mL
Thyroxine (T4), serum	
Total	5–12 pg/dL
Free	0.9–2.4 ng/dL

Free T4 index	4–11
Triodothyronine, resin (T3)	25%–35%
Triiodothyronine, serum (T3)	70–195 ng/dL
Vitamin D	
1,25-dihydroxy, serum	25–65 pg/mL
25-hydroxy, serum	15–80 ng/mL

Gastrointestinal

Fecal urobilinogen	40–280 mg/24 h
Gastrin, serum	0–180 pg/mL
Lactose tolerance test	Increase in plasma glucose: >15 mg/dL
Lipase, ascitic fluid	<200 U/L
Secretin-cholecystokinin pancreatic function	>80 meq/L of HCO_3 in at least 1 specimen collected over 1 h
Stool fat	<5 g/d on a 100-g fat diet
Stool nitrogen	<2 g/d
Stool weight	<200 g/d

Hematology

Activated partial thromboplastin time	25–35 s
Bleeding time	<10 min
Coagulation factors, plasma	
Factor I	150–350 mg/dL
Factor II	60%–150% of normal
Factor V	60%–150% of normal
Factor VII	60%–150% of normal
Factor VIII	60%–150% of normal
Factor IX	60%–150% of normal
Factor X	60%–150% of normal
Factor XI	60%–150% of normal
Factor XII	60%–150% of normal
Erythrocyte count	4.2–5.9 million cells/μL
Erythropoietin	<30 mU/mL
D-dimer	<0.5 μg/mL
Ferritin, serum	15–200 ng/mL
Glucose-6-phosphate dehydrogenase, blood	5–15 U/g Hgb
Haptoglobin, serum	50–150 mg/dL
Hematocrit	
Male	41%–51%
Female	36%–47%

Hemoglobin, blood	
Male	14–17 g/dL
Female	12–16 g/dL
Hemoglobin, plasma	0.5–5 mg/dL
Leukocyte alkaline phosphatase	15–40 mg of phosphorus liberated/h per 10^{10} cells
Score	13–130/100 polymorphonuclear neutrophils and band forms
Leukocyte count	
Nonblacks	4000–10,000/μL
Blacks	3500–10,000/μL
Lymphocytes	
CD4+ cell count	640–1175/μL
CD8+ cell count	335–875/μL
CD4:CD8 ratio	1.0–4.0
Mean corpuscular hemoglobin (MCH)	28–32 pg
Mean corpuscular hemoglobin concentration (MCHC)	32–36 g/dL
Mean corpuscular volume (MCV)	80–100 fL
Platelet count	150,000–350,000/μL
Protein C activity, plasma	67%–131%
Protein C resistance	2.2–2.6
Protein S activity, plasma	82%–144%
Prothrombin time	11–13 s
Reticulocyte count	0.5%–1.5% of erythrocytes
Absolute	23,000–90,000 cells/μL
Schilling test (oral administration of radioactive cobalamin-labeled vitamin B_{12})	8.5%–28% excreted in urine per 24–48 h
Sedimentation rate, erythrocyte (Westergren)	
Male	0–15 mm/h
Female	0–20 mm/h
Volume, blood	
Plasma	
Male	25–44 mL/kg body weight
Female	28–43 mL/kg body weight
Erythrocyte	
Male	25–35 mL/kg body weight
Female	20–30 mL/kg body weight

Urine

Amino acids	200–400 mg/24 h
Amylase	6.5–48.1 U/h
Calcium	100–300 mg/d on unrestricted diet
Chloride	80–250 meq/d (varies with intake)
Copper	0–100 µg/24 h
Creatine	
Male	4–40 mg/24 h
Female	0–100 mg/24 h
Creatinine	15–25 mg/kg per 24 h
Creatinine clearance	90–140 mL/min
Osmolality	38–1400 mosm/kg H_2O
Phosphate, tubular resorption	79%–94% (0.79–0.94) of filtered load
Potassium	25–100 meq/24 h (varies with intake)
Protein	<100 mg/24 h
Sodium	100–260 meq/24 h (varies with intake)
Uric acid	250–750 mg/24 h (varies with diet)
Urobilinogen	0.05–2.5 mg/24 h

S **What is the quality of the patient's chest pain?**
Common descriptions of angina include:

- Pressure
- Tightness
- Band-like constriction

- Heaviness
- Discomfort
- Weight on the chest

Fleeting, sharp, or stabbing pains are less commonly associated with angina.
Burning pain is often a symptom of gastroesophageal reflux disease (GERD).
Severe, tearing pain may signify aortic dissection rather than angina.
Pleuritic pain (pain with inspiration) is more suggestive of pulmonary disease
  (pneumonia, pulmonary embolism/infarction) or pericarditis, than of ischemia.

Where is the pain located?
Ischemic chest pain is poorly localized but often described as substernal. It may also
  present as epigastric.
Pain that can be pinpointed with certainty is often musculoskeletal and unlikely to
  be anginal.
Pain localized to the right precordium is also less likely angina.

Does the pain radiate anywhere?
Radiation to the neck, jaw, or arm is a classic feature of angina.
Radiation to the back may indicate aortic dissection.
Radiation to the left shoulder suggests a diaphragmatic process

Are there aggravating or alleviating factors?
Pain coming on with exertion and relieved by rest is typical of angina.
Pain that is worse when supine and improved when sitting forward is a feature of
  pericarditis.
Pain reproducible with palpation over the affected area is often musculoskeletal in
  origin.
Aggravation by eating is a feature of peptic ulcer disease or GERD.

Are there any associated features?
Angina is often associated with nausea, vomiting, or dyspnea.
Fever or hemoptysis may be indicative of pneumonia or pulmonary emboli.
Water brash often occurs with GERD.
Dyspnea may be present with angina, myocardial infarction, pneumonia, pulmonary
  embolism (PE), pneumothorax.

Obtain a medical history
Certain risk factors may be associated with particular causes of chest pain.
Risk factors for angina include hypertension, diabetes mellitus, smoking, dyslipi-
  demia, and a positive family history.

- Hypertension is also a risk factor for aortic dissection.

A period of immobility (e.g., bed rest or air travel) is a risk factor for deep venous
  thrombosis and pulmonary emboli.
Trauma predisposes to rib fractures and pneumothorax.

 Check vital signs
Patients with angina are often tachycardic and hypertensive.
Patients with aortic dissections may be hypertensive (descending dissections) or
  hypotensive (ascending dissections), and often have asymmetric pulses and
  blood pressure in their arms.
Patients with pneumonia or PE are often tachycardic and hypoxic.

Perform a directed physical examination
Aortic dissection may be associated with an aortic insufficiency murmur and asymmetric pulses and blood pressure.
Pericarditis is associated with a pericardial friction rub.
Musculoskeletal pain (e.g., costochondritis) may be reproducible by chest palpation.
Pulmonary emboli/infarct may be associated with a pleural rub.
Pneumonia is associated with focal rhonchi in the involved lung field.
Herpes zoster is associated with a dermatomal rash in the involved area.

Chest pain

Differential diagnosis

- Angina	- Aortic dissection
- Myocardial infarction	- Pulmonary emboli
- Pericarditis	- Pneumonia
- GERD	- Musculoskeletal chest pain
- Esophageal spasm	- Chest wall trauma (rib fracture)

P **Obtain an electrocardiogram**
Angina and myocardial infarction are associated with dynamic ST segment abnormalities during the pain.
PE may be associated with an S wave in lead I, and a Q wave and T wave inversion in lead III (S1Q3T3 pattern).
Pericarditis is associated with PR segment depression and diffuse ST segment elevation.

Obtain a chest x-ray
Look for focal infiltrates (pneumonia), peripheral wedge-shaped infiltrates (PE), wide mediastinum (aortic dissection), pneumothorax, rib fractures.

Perform further testing depending on the suspected diagnosis
Aortic dissection: transesophageal echocardiography, chest CT, chest MRI.
Myocardial infarction: serial cardiac enzymes and electrocardiogramy (ECG); cardiac catheterization for patients with STEMI.
Angina: exercise stress testing.
Pulmonary embolism: V/Q scan, CT angiogram, pulmonary angiography.
Pericarditis: serial ECG and physical examinations; echocardiogram.
GERD: upper GI series, trial of proton pump inhibitors.
Esophageal spasm: esophageal manometry.

Institute specific treatment based on the results of the diagnostic studies

S **Was the onset of dyspnea sudden, gradual, or chronic?**
Sudden dyspnea may occur with angina, acute congestive heart failure (CHF), pulmonary embolism (PE), pneumothorax.
Gradual dyspnea may occur with chronic CHF, chronic obstructive pulmonary disease (COPD), pneumonia, pleural effusions.
Chronic dyspnea may occur with COPD, chronic CHF, interstitial lung disease.

Does the patient experience dyspnea at rest or with exertion?
Dyspnea on exertion may occur with most causes of dyspnea.
Dyspnea at rest suggests advanced cardiac or pulmonary disease.

Is the dyspnea worse when lying down?
Orthopnea is usually due to cardiac disease but is occasionally caused by lung disease.
Paroxysmal nocturnal dyspnea is characteristic of CHF.

Is the dyspnea associated with other symptoms?
Concomitant chest pain occurs with angina, myocardial infarction (MI), PE, pneumothorax, pneumonia.
 • Dyspnea and pleuritic chest pain suggest PE.
Concomitant hemoptysis occurs with PE, pneumonia.
Cough or wheezing occurs with COPD, pneumonia; occasionally with CHF.

Is there associated anxiety or panic?
Suggests anxiety disorder.

 Review the patient's vital signs
Dyspnea is often associated with tachypnea and deceased oxygen saturation.
Check ambulatory oxygen saturation.

Perform a physical examination looking for the following features
Skin color:
 • Pale skin suggests anemia.
 • Peripheral cyanosis suggests hypoxemia.
Look for signs of heart failure:
 • Elevated JVP • Edema • Third or fourth heart sound
Listen for mitral or aortic valve murmurs.
Perform a thorough pulmonary examination:
 • Wheezing suggests COPD.
 • Bilateral crackles suggest CHF or interstitial lung disease.
 • A focal area of crackles suggests pneumonia.
 • Decreased breath sounds and dullness to percussion suggests a pleural effusion.
 • Asymmetric breath sounds suggests pneumothorax, pneumonia, pleural effusion.

Obtain a medical history
| - Coronary artery disease | - Hypertension | - Cardiomyopathy |
| - Asthma | - COPD | - Interstitial lung disease |

Obtain a social history
Obtain a detailed smoking history.
Review possible toxic exposures at work or home.

A

Dyspnea
Dyspnea is the unpleasant, subjective awareness of respiration. May be described differently by different people.

- Tightness
- Air hunger
- Shortness of breath
- Shallow breathing
- Suffocation

Differential diagnosis
Primary pulmonary disorders

- Asthma, COPD
- Pulmonary hypertension
- Pulmonary embolus
- Aspiration
- Infection (pneumonia, bronchitis)
- Interstitial lung disease
- Pneumothorax
- Anaphylaxis

Cardiac disorders

- Acute ischemia
- Valvular heart disease
- Arrhythmia
- Congestive heart failure
- Pericardial effusion

Other

- Anxiety/panic disorder
- Anemia
- Acidosis

P

Stabilize the patient's respiratory status
Supplemental oxygen by face mask or nasal cannula to maintain oxygen saturation >92%. Treat respiratory failure with mechanical ventilation.
Consider use of morphine to blunt the sensation of dyspnea.

Obtain a chest x-ray
Hyperinflation and flattened diaphragms suggest asthma or COPD.
CHF may cause cardiomegaly, vascular engorgement, Kerley B lines, cephalization of vessels, and pulmonary edema.
Lobar or more diffuse consolidation suggests pneumonia.
Cardiomegaly may indicate LV systolic dysfunction, valvular disease, or pericardial effusion.

Obtain an electrocardiogram (during period of symptoms if possible):
Examine for signs of ischemia, arrhythmias, acute right heart strain ($S_1Q_3T_3$), ventricular hypertrophy, or atrial enlargement.

Obtain basic laboratories
CBC to exclude anemia; chemistries to exclude acidosis, renal failure, or hyperglycemia.

Consider obtaining a brain natriuretic peptide (BNP)
BNP is secreted by the ventricles in response to increased pressure.
- Elevated (usually >400 pg/mL) in CHF but normal (<100 pg/mL) in pure lung disease.

Consider obtaining an arterial blood gas
Can accurately assess the degree of hypoxemia.

Perform specific testing depending on suspected diagnosis
Obtain a ventilation-perfusion scan or CT angiogram in patients with suspected PE.
Obtain an echocardiogram in patients with suspected cardiac disease.

Consider pulmonary function tests to evaluate for obstructive or restrictive lung disease

Consider assessing hemodynamics with a pulmonary arterial catheter if cause of dyspnea remains uncertain
Can accurately differentiate cardiac and pulmonary causes of dyspnea.

Institute specific treatments depending on the specific cause of the dyspnea identified

S **What is the pattern of the palpitations?**
Rapid, regular palpitations suggest sinus tachycardia, supraventricular tachycardia (SVT), or ventricular tachycardia (VT).
Rapid irregular palpitations suggest atrial fibrillation.
Single palpitations or "skipped beats" suggest premature atrial or ventricular contractions.
Slow, pounding palpitations suggest sinus bradycardia or heart block.
Patients can often mimic the palpitations by tapping their fingers on a table.

Do the palpitations begin and end suddenly or gradually?
Palpitations that start and stop suddenly suggest SVT or VT.
Palpitations that gradually speed up and slow down suggest sinus tachycardia.

Are there associated symptoms?
- Lightheadedness	- Dizziness	- Presyncope
- Syncope	- Chest pain	- Dyspnea

Is there anything that precipitates the palpitations?
Palpitations that occur with exertion/exercise suggest sinus tachycardia.
Rarely, VT may be precipitated by exercise.

Can the patient stop the palpitations in any way?
Termination of palpitations with vagal maneuvers (e.g., Valsalva maneuver, gagging, coughing) suggests AV nodal reentrant tachycardia or AV reentrant tachycardia.

Does the patient have a history of heart disease?
Valvular heart disease is often associated with SVT.
Ischemic heart disease is often associated with VT.

Does the patient have other medical conditions that predispose to palpitations?
- Thyroid disease	- Chronic obstructive pulmonary disease
- Anxiety or panic disorder	- Anemia
- Hypertension	- Pregnancy

Obtain a full medications history including prescription, nonprescription, and illicit drugs that may cause palpitations
- Beta-agonist inhalers	- Theophylline	- Over-the-counter
- Herbal supplements	- Caffeine	cold remedies
- Nicotine	- Alcohol	- Cocaine
- Antiarrhythmic agents	- Antipsychotic agents	- Weight loss drugs

O **Review the patient's vital signs**

Feel the pulse for 30 to 60 seconds
Feel for heart rate and rhythm.

Perform a physical examination looking for the following features
Signs of hyperthyroidism (e.g., lid lag, exophthalmos, tremor, hyperreflexivity).
Thyroid goiter.
Cardiac murmurs including the click of mitral valve prolapse.
Evidence of a cardiomyopathy (displaced point of maximal impulse, S_3, elevated jugular venous pressure).
Evidence of anemia.

Palpitations
Palpitations are the conscious awareness of the heart beat and usually result from an abnormal heart rate or rhythm.

Differential diagnosis
Arrhythmias
- Sinus tachycardia
- Ventricular tachycardia
- Bradycardia

- Supraventricular tachycardia
- Premature atrial or ventricular contractions
- Heart block

Mitral valve prolapse syndrome
Psychiatric conditions
- Anxiety

- Panic disorder

 Obtain an electrocardiogram
If obtained during period of symptoms it may be diagnostic of a specific arrhythmia.
- A normal electrocardiogram (ECG) during periods of palpitations makes a cardiac cause of palpitations unlikely.

May reveal evidence of structural or functional heart disease even if obtained when the patient is asymptomatic.
- Prior myocardial infarction
- Ventricular hypertrophy
- Atrial enlargement
- Conduction abnormality
- Short PR interval and a delta wave (Wolff-Parkinson-White syndrome)
- Prolonged QT interval

Obtain basic laboratories
- Complete blood cell count
- Thyroid function tests

- Serum electrolyte panel
- Toxicology screen (if drug use suspected)

Perform prolonged ECG monitoring if arrhythmia not present on ECG
24-hour Holter monitor if palpitations occur frequently.
- Records every heartbeat for 24 hours.

30-day event monitor if palpitations are infrequent.
- Records the rhythm for a brief time when activated by the patient at the time of symptoms.

Implantable monitor for very infrequent events.
- Implanted in the chest wall and can be left in place for years.

Consider obtaining an echocardiogram if structural heart disease is suspected

Consider performing electrophysiologic studies (rarely required)
Consider if recurrent undiagnosed palpitations and high risk of malignant arrhythmia.
- Prior myocardial infarction
- Syncope with palpitations
- Family history of sudden death

Educate patient on avoidance of caffeine, alcohol, and other triggering factors

Institute specific treatment depending on the identified cause of the palpitations

S **Did the patient truly have loss of consciousness?**
True syncope implies a temporary loss of consciousness and should be distinguished from lightheadedness, dizziness, or presyncope.

Did the patient have any symptoms that preceded the syncopal event?
Preceding nausea or diaphoresis suggests *vasovagal syncope.*
Preceding palpitations suggest an *arrhythmia* (usually ventricular tachycardia [VT] or a bradyarrhythmia).
  • Supraventricular tachycardia (SVT) rarely causes syncope in the absence of structural heart disease or a bypass tract.
Chest pain suggests myocardial ischemia, aortic dissection, pulmonary embolism.
Sudden loss of consciousness without warning symptoms suggests an *arrhythmia.*

What was the patient doing at the time of the syncopal event?
Syncope during exertion suggests *obstructive cardiac disease* (aortic or mitral stenosis, hypertrophic cardiomyopathy, or pulmonary hypertension).
Syncope following a painful or emotional stimulus suggests a *vasovagal reaction.*
Syncope immediately after standing suggests *orthostatic hypotension.*
Syncope after prolonged standing suggests *neurocardiogenic syncope.*
Syncope during urination, defecation or cough suggests *situational syncope.*
Syncope when looking upward suggests *vertebrobasilar insufficiency,* while syncope after looking to one side suggests *carotid sinus hypersensitivity.*

Did the patient bite his or her tongue or have urinary incontinence during the event?
These symptoms suggest seizure, not syncope.

Does the patient have any condition that may predispose to syncope?
Coronary artery disease or congestive heart failure.
  • Both predispose to cardiac arrhythmias, especially in patients with depressed left ventricular ejection fraction.
Diabetes and Parkinson's disease predispose to autonomic dysfunction.
Prior cerebrovascular accident (CVA) or head trauma may predispose to seizure.

Is the patient on medications that predispose to syncope?
Beta-blockers or calcium channel blockers may cause bradycardia or heart block.
Most antihypertensive agents can cause orthostatic syncope.
Diuretics may cause volume depletion and orthostasis.
Many anti-arrhythmic agents have pro-arrhythmic effects.
Tricyclic antidepressants, antifungal agents, and antihistamines may cause VT.

Did anyone witness the syncopal event?
Patient may have no recall of the events – history must be elicited from witnesses.

O **Review vital signs including orthostatic pulse and blood pressure**

Perform focused physical examination, looking for
Evidence of volume depletion.
Evidence of heart failure.
Carotid and/or vertebral bruits.
Murmur of aortic or mitral stenosis or hypertrophic obstructive cardiomyopathy.
Focal neurologic deficits.

Perform carotid sinus massage if history suggestive of carotid sinus hypersensitivity
Should not be performed if the patient has a carotid bruit or a history of CVA or transient ischemic attack (TIA).

Obtain an electrocardiogram, looking for
- Bradycardia
- Tachyarrhythmias
- Prolonged QT interval
- Heart block
- Prior myocardial infarction
- Short PR interval and a delta wave (Wolff-Parkinson-White syndrome)

Obtain complete blood cell count and electrolyte panel
Exclude anemia, hypo-or hyperkalemia, hypomagnesemia, and hypocalcemia.

Syncope
The transient loss of consciousness and postural tone resulting from inadequate cerebral perfusion. The onset is sudden and recovery is usually abrupt and complete.

Differential diagnosis
- Seizure
- Hypoglycemia
- Pseudoseizure
- CVA/TIA

Prognosis
Cardiovascular syncope is associated with a 30% 1-year mortality.
Vasovagal (including orthostatic) syncope has no increased risk of death.

Admit the patient to a telemetry floor if a cardiac cause of syncope is suspected

Treat reversible causes of syncope
Give IV fluids if dehydrated, stop offending medications, correct electrolyte abnormalities.

Obtain further diagnostic studies depending on suspected cause
If history is consistent with a vasovagal episode, orthostatic hypotension, or situational syncope, no further work-up is usually needed.
If history or examination suggests underlying structural heart disease, an *echocardiogram* should be obtained.
Patients with depressed left ventricular (LV) ejection fraction have a worse prognosis.
If history suggests an arrhythmia and LV function is normal, consider prolonged monitoring with a *Holter monitor* (24 hours) or an *event recorder* (1 month).
If history suggests an arrhythmia and LV function is depressed, consider referral for electrophysiologic study.
If ischemia suspected, consider stress testing versus cardiac catheterization.
If neurocardiogenic syncope suspected, consider *Upright Tilt Table Test*
- May induce bradycardia (cardioinhibitory response), hypotension (vasodepressor response), and syncope in susceptible people.
Electroencephalography, brain computed tomography or magnetic resonance imaging, and carotid Doppler ultrasound may be indicated if seizure, CVA, or TIA suspected.

Begin specific treatments depending on specific cause of syncope identified
If ventricular tachyarrhythmia is identified, consider implantable cardioverter/defibrillator placement.
If supraventricular tachyarrhythmia thought to be the cause, treat with rate-lowering medications, antiarrhythmic agents, or radiofrequency ablation.
Symptomatic bradyarrhythmias require placement of a permanent pacemaker unless a reversible cause identified (e.g., medication effect).
Ischemia may be managed with anti-ischemic drugs or coronary revascularization.
Symptomatic aortic or mitral stenosis usually requires valve replacement surgery.
Neurocardiogenic syncope often responds to treatment with beta-blockers.

S Has the patient been effectively resuscitated?

If the patient has no pulse or blood pressure, continue resuscitation using advanced cardiac life support protocols until patient has stabilized.

How long after cardiac arrest was resuscitation started and circulation restored?

Cardiopulmonary resuscitation (CPR) should be started immediately and defibrillation should occur within 4 minutes of arrest. Prognosis worsens significantly with longer response times.

Did the patient have any symptoms that preceded the cardiac arrest?

Survivors of sudden cardiac death (SCD) are often initially neurologically impaired and unable to provide any history. Relatives or witnesses should be sought and questioned.

Preceding chest pain suggests an acute ischemic event.

Progressive dyspnea for several hours or days suggests decompensated congestive heart failure (CHF).

Chronic dyspnea on exertion, pedal edema, orthopnea suggest cardiomyopathy.

• Cardiomyopathy, with or without coronary artery disease, is a major risk factor for SCD.

Sudden loss of consciousness without premonitory symptoms suggests ventricular tachycardia/ventricular fibrillation.

Palpitations suggest a tachyarrhythmia. Bradycardia causing SCD is uncommon.

Does the patient have a history of cardiac disease?

- Aortic stenosis   - Dilated cardiomyopathy
- Prior syncope   - Hypertrophic cardiomyopathy
- Bypass tract (Wolff-Parkinson-White syndrome [WPW])
- Coronary artery disease (~70% of SCD patients have an acute or prior myocardial infarction)

Is there any family history of sudden cardiac death?

Consider familial cardiomyopathies or long QT syndrome.

Is the patient on medications that predispose to arrhythmias?

May prolong the QT interval and predispose to polymorphic VT (*Torsade*).

Antiarrhythmic agents (quinidine, procainamide, sotalol, disopyramide).

Antimicrobial agents (erythromycin, pentamidine, quinolones, antifungals).

Antipsychotic agents (chlorpromazine, haloperidol, thioridazine).

O Check the vital signs including oxygen saturation

Perform a rapid cardiovascular examination

Listen for significant murmurs (e.g., aortic stenosis).

Assess for evidence of CHF (elevated jugular venous pressure, S_3 gallop, pulmonary rales).

Perform a neurologic examination

Assess mental status.

Assess cranial nerve function (corneal and pupillary reflex, gag reflex, etc).

Check for intentional movement of each extremity.

Obtain a 12-lead electrocardiogram

Look for evidence of active ischemia (ST elevation or depression).

Look for evidence of prior infarction (Q wave, T wave inversions).

Assess for conduction disease – closely examine PR, QRS, and QT interval.

Short PR, especially with a "delta" wave, suggests WPW.

Request an electrolyte panel
Acid-base disorders and abnormalities of potassium, magnesium, and calcium can precipitate arrhythmias.

Sudden cardiac death
Sudden and unexpected death from a natural cardiac cause, usually within 1 hour of the onset of symptoms. Immediate CPR and defibrillation may result in recovery, with patients then being deemed "survivors of sudden cardiac death."

Etiology
Ischemic heart disease (65%–70%).
Other structural heart disease (10%).
 • Hypertrophic or dilated cardiomyopathy, valve disease, aortic dissection.
Primary arrhythmia in the absence of structural heart disease (5%–10%).
 • WPW, long-QT syndrome, Bruggada syndrome, electrolyte abnormalities.
Noncardiac causes (10%–20%).
 • Trauma, PE, airway obstruction, bleeding.

Stabilize the respiratory status
Intubation and ventilation are often required.

Stabilize blood pressure if hypotensive
Give empiric fluid bolus (250 cc saline) if without pulmonary congestion.
Start dopamine as needed for hypotension—monitor for recurrent arrhythmias.

Perform emergent cardiac catheterization and revascularization if postresuscitation electrocardiogram (ECG) reveals ischemic ST depressions or ST elevations
Avoid in patients with prolonged arrest and no neurologic function.
Consider elective catheterization for patients without ischemia on ECG.

Admit to the intensive care unit

Obtain a cardiology consult

Obtain an echocardiogram (immediately)
Quantify left ventricular and right ventricular function, assess valves, and evaluate for pericardial tamponade and proximal aortic dissection.

Institute hypothermic therapy (within 6 hours of resuscitation) in patients without spontaneous neurologic recovery
Cool to approximately 94°F for 24 hours with cooling blankets or intravenous device.
Requires pharmacologic paralysis and sedation to avoid shivering.
Contraindicated if systolic blood pressure less than 90 mm Hg, coagulopathy, infection, electrolyte disorder.
Improves neurologic outcomes and functional level.

Check serial cardiac enzymes and treat any predisposing factors
Discontinue medications that prolong the QT interval.
Correct acid-base and electrolyte disorders.

Perform serial neurologic examinations
The absence of pupillary or corneal reflexes at 24 hours and the absence of motor function at 72 hours are poor prognostic signs.
Perform head computed tomography if focal neurologic deficits are present.
Consult neurology if no significant improvement after 24 to 48 hours.

Consider electrophysiologic study and/or implantation of a cardioverter/defibrillator in all SCD survivors with intact neurologic function

S **What are the patient's symptoms?**

Most patients with variant angina present with severe substernal chest pain.
- May be identical in quality to angina pectoris (see SOAP 7), but tends to occur in a younger age group, in patients with fewer cardiac risk factors, and is more common in women.

Patients may also present with ventricular arrhythmias or sudden cardiac death.

What precipitates the patient's symptoms?

Variant angina usually occurs at rest, rarely with exertion.
- Occurs more commonly between midnight and early morning.

May be precipitated by smoking or hyperventilation.

Does the patient have a history of other vasospastic disorders?

Patients with variant angina often have migraines and Raynaud's phenomena.

Does the patient have a history of substance abuse?

Cocaine can precipitate coronary vasospasm in patients with or without coronary artery disease (CAD).

Tobacco smoking is a risk factor for variant angina.

Perform a review of systems

May suggest an alternative diagnosis (e.g., pericarditis, myocarditis, aortic dissection).

O **Check vital signs**

Hypotension and tachyarrhythmias can occur during episodes.

Perform a physical examination

Cardiac: may be normal in the absence of ischemia. An S_3, S_4, or transient murmur of mitral regurgitation may be heard during episodes.

Vascular bruits: diminished pulses and vascular bruits indicate atherosclerotic vascular disease and increase the likelihood of concomitant CAD.

Skin: Look for changes in the fingers consistent with Raynaud's disease.

Obtain an electrocardiogram

Vasospastic angina is characterized by transient ST segment elevation during chest pain episodes.
- In typical angina, chest pain is associated with transient ST depression.

Transient heart block may occur with vasospasm of the right coronary artery.

Ventricular arrhythmias may occur with vasospasm of the left coronary artery.

Send serum for serial cardiac enzymes

Most episodes of coronary vasospasm do not lead to myocardial infarction; however, it can occur with prolonged episodes.

Prinzmetal's (variant) angina
A syndrome of anginal chest pain that occurs almost exclusively at rest, and is associated with ST segment elevation on ECG.

Pathophysiology
Occurs secondary to coronary vasospasm as opposed to the acute plaque rupture seen with coronary artery disease. The vasospasm can occur in normal coronary arteries (pure vasospasm) or in areas adjacent to atheromatous plaque (Prinzmetal's angina), and involves both the large epicardial arteries and the microvasculature.

Differential diagnosis
- Myocardial infarction secondary to coronary artery disease
- Aortic dissection with coronary occlusion
- Myocarditis
- Pericarditis

Admit to a monitored or intensive care unit bed

Administer acute vasodilator therapy
Nitroglycerin (NTG) sublingually or IV.
Short-acting calcium channel blockers such as nifedipine, diltiazem, or verapamil can also be used.
Consider use of morphine sulphate for its pain relief and vasodilatory properties if required.

Obtain cardiology consult for patients with persistent chest pain despite vasodilators
Consider cardiac catheterization.
● In patients with persistent chest pain and ischemic electrocardiogram (ECG) changes.
● In patients in whom the diagnosis is uncertain.
◆ May see spontaneous vasospasm during cardiac catheterization.
◆ Can provoke vasospasm by hyperventilation or by infusion of acetylcholine or ergonovine into the coronary arteries.

If the diagnosis of vasospastic angina is confirmed, percutaneous coronary intervention should be avoided as it has the potential to provoke further vasospasm.

Institute chronic vasodilator therapy
Long-acting calcium channel blockers (e.g., nifedipine 30–90 mg/day, diltiazem 120–480 mg/day) are very effective at preventing recurrent episodes of vasospasm.
Long-acting nitrates are also effective.
In patients with persistent symptoms, the addition of an alpha-adrenergic blocker may be beneficial.

Nonselective beta-blockers should be avoided as they can aggravate vasospasm.

Consider surgical plexectomy or sympathectomy for patients who are refractory to all medical therapies

Pursue aggressive risk factor modification
- Smoking cessation
- Diabetes control
- Abstinence from cocaine
- Lipid lowering therapy
- Hypertension control
- Weight reduction

S **What is the patient's anginal symptom?**
Chest pain is the most common anginal symptom.
Dyspnea, nausea, arm pain may be "anginal equivalents."

Is the patient's chest pain consistent with angina?
Anginal pain is usually characterized by:
- A "pressure," "heaviness," "squeezing," or vague "discomfort."
- Located substernal or over the left chest.
- Precipitated by stress (physical or emotional).
- Lasts 5–10 minutes.
- Relieved with rest or after the use of nitroglycerin.

Dull, sharp, or stabbing pain lasting for only a few seconds or for several hours consecutively is unlikely to be angina.

Are there other symptoms associated with the chest pain?
Angina is frequently associated with dyspnea, diaphoresis, and/or nausea.

Does the chest pain radiate anywhere?
Anginal chest pain may radiate to the left neck, jaw, shoulder, or arm.
Angina does not usually radiate to the back or abdomen.

Has there been a recent change in the pattern or character of the patient's angina?
A significant increase in the frequency, duration, or severity of the angina or new onset of rest angina is considered unstable. (See SOAP 8.)
How much exertion does it take to precipitate the patient's angina?
- Is this a change from a prior pattern?
- Is the angina occurring with less exertion?

Does the patient have a prior history of coronary artery disease?
Is the current symptom similar to the prior angina?
Has the patient had prior cardiac tests (stress tests, echocardiogram, catheterization)?

Obtain a medical history including risk factors for cardiac disease
Hypertension
Dyslipidemia
Tobacco use
Diabetes mellitus (considered a coronary artery disease [CAD] equivalent by current guidelines)
Family history of premature CAD (Male <55 years, Female <60 years)
Peripheral or cerebrovascular disease

 Check vital signs

Perform a focused cardiovascular examination
Assess jugular venous pressure.
Auscultate for murmurs and additional heart sounds (S_3 or S_4).
Listen for carotid and femoral arterial bruits.
- Cerebrovascular and peripheral vascular disease often coexists with CAD.
Assess for signs of heart failure.
- Pulmonary rales, pedal edema, elevated JVP.

Review the patient's electrocardiogram
Look for evidence of prior infarction, assess for left ventricular hypertrophy.

Stable angina

Angina that occurs in a stable, predictable pattern. May be a chronic syndrome in patients with known CAD or may be the presenting pattern of a patient with previously undiagnosed CAD.

Pathophysiology

Usually results from a fixed narrowing of a coronary artery by atherosclerotic plaque.
- A 70% stenosis of a coronary artery may cause exertional angina.
- A 90% stenosis of a coronary artery may cause angina at rest.

May result from excessive myocardial demand without CAD (anemia, tachycardia).

Differential diagnosis

Rarely confused with unstable angina, myocardial infarction, pericarditis, aortic dissection, or pulmonary embolism.

Needs to be differentiated from noncardiac chest pain (GERD, esophageal spasm, peptic ulcer disease, musculoskeletal chest pain, anxiety).

 Start antianginal medication if the history is diagnostic of angina

All patients should be started on aspirin 81 mg daily.

Choice of other agents is left to physician preference—consider comorbid conditions, side effect profiles, etc.
- Beta-blockers (e.g., metoprolol 25 mg bid, atenolol 25 mg qd)
- Calcium channel blockers (e.g., diltiazem 120 mg qd, verapamil 120 mg qd)
- Nitrates (e.g., isosorbide dinitrate 10 mg tid, isosorbide mononitrate 30 mg qd)

Anti-anginal medications should be started at low to moderate dose and titrated based on the heart rate (HR) and blood pressure (BP) response.
- The ideal BP in patients with stable angina is less than 125/85 mm Hg.
- The ideal resting HR in patients with stable angina ~60–70 beats per minute.

Give the patient a prescription for sublingual NTG with instructions on its use.

Check a complete blood cell count and electrolytes

Exclude anemia as a contributing factor to presenting symptoms.

Thrombocytopenia and abnormalities in renal function may impact medical therapy.

Obtain a fasting lipid profile

Treat based on recent guidelines. (See SOAP 58.)

Consider stress testing

As a diagnostic test if the patient's symptoms are not clearly anginal.
- Withhold beta-blockers or calcium channel blockers for 12 hours before study to allow the patient to reach an adequate HR.

As a prognostic test in patients with presumed angina/CAD.

Treat modifiable risk factors

Hypertension—goal BP <125/85 mg Hg.

Diabetes—Check fasting glucose, hemoglobin A1c. Tight glycemic control is imperative.

Smoking cessation.

Encourage weight loss as needed.

Prescribe an exercise regimen—may benefit from cardiac rehab.

Consider further testing based on clinical findings

Echocardiogram if left ventricular dysfunction suspected (e.g., evidence of congestive heart failure).

Vascular studies if symptoms (claudication, transient ischemic attack) or vascular bruits present.

S **What was the patient's presenting symptom?**

Chest pain (angina) is the most common presenting symptom of unstable angina (UA) or non–ST-segment elevation myocardial infarction (NSTEMI).
Other common presenting symptoms/syndromes include:

- Shortness of breath
- Heart failure
- Nausea, vomiting
- Arrhythmias (including ventricular tachycardia)

What was the pattern of the patient's angina?

Angina is considered "unstable" if it occurs in one of several patterns:

- New onset angina brought on by minimal exertion.
- Crescendo angina (increasing in severity) on a background of stable angina.
- Rest angina unresponsive to sublingual nitroglycerin use or of greater than 20 minutes duration.

Does the patient have high-risk clinical features?

- Age older than 65
- On aspirin therapy
- Ongoing chest pain
- ST segment changes during chest pain
- Previous coronary artery disease (myocardial infarction [MI], percutaneous coronary intervention)

Does the patient have risk factors for coronary artery disease?

Obtain a medical history

Obtain a thorough review of systems

May suggest other causes of the chest pain (e.g., aortic dissection, pericarditis, etc).

O **Check vital signs**

Hypertension and tachycardia can exacerbate ischemia.

Perform a physical examination looking for the following features

An S_3 or S_4 on cardiac auscultation may be present during ischemia.
A new or transient mitral regurgitation murmur may indicate ischemic papillary muscle dysfunction.
Evidence of heart failure (e.g., pulmonary rales, pleural effusion, elevated jugular venous pressure).

- Congestive heart failure occurring during unstable angina or a NSTEMI usually indicates either significant myocardial ischemia or pre-existing left ventricular dysfunction.

Obtain an electrocardiogram

ST segment depressions are a marker of high risk.
Attempt to obtain an old electrocardiogram (ECG) to compare for subtle changes.
Serial ECGs should be obtained to evaluate for evolutionary changes of a MI and to ensure that ischemic ST changes return to baseline after the angina resolves.

Obtain serial cardiac enzymes (creatinine kinase [CK], and troponin)

Will be elevated with NSTEMI but not with UA.
Obtain every 6 hours three times, or until the CK level peaks.
CK—increases by ~6 hours after a MI, peaks at 24 hours, and returns to normal in 2–3 days.

- The peak level of CK correlates with the extent of myocardial necrosis.

Cardiac troponin—highly sensitive marker, begins to increase ~3–6 hours after a MI, peaks in 24 hours, and remains elevated for 10–14 days.

- Very useful for diagnosing a MI that occurred several days previously.

Request complete blood cell count and electrolytes

Anemia can exacerbate symptoms.
Thrombocytopenia will affect use of antiplatelet agents and heparin.
Keep potassium greater than 4.0 and magnesium greater than 2.0 to decrease potential of arrhythmia.

A Unstable angina and non–ST segment elevation myocardial infarction

Generally reflects rupture of an atherosclerotic plaque resulting in partial thrombosis of a coronary artery, impaired coronary blood flow, and resultant myocardial ischemia or infarction.

NSTEMI is differentiated from UA by the presence of elevated cardiac enzymes.

Differential diagnosis
- ST elevation MI (See SOAP 9)
- Pulmonary embolus
- Pericarditis
- Gastroesophageal reflux disease
- Stable angina
- Myocarditis
- Aortic dissection
- Musculoskeletal chest pain

P Admit to a monitored floor (coronary care unit or telemetry unit)

Initiate the following therapy immediately
Aspirin 325 mg daily (the first dose should be chewed).
Nitroglycerin sublingually or as an intravenous drip to control anginal symptoms.
Morphine sulphate as required.
Supplemental oxygen.
Low-molecular-weight or unfractionated heparin as an anti-thrombotic agent.
Beta-blocking agent for its anti-ischemic and anti-arrhythmic properties.
  ● Metoprolol 25 mg four times daily for first 24 hours, then twice daily.
Consider giving loading dose of clopidogrel (300 mg orally) if high suspicion of need for percutaneous coronary revascularization.

Calculate the TIMI risk score by assigning a value of I to each of the following criteria
- Age greater than 65
- ST segment deviation on the ECG
- Prior coronary stenosis of 50% or more
- At least three risk factors for CAD
- At least two anginal events in the prior 24 hours
- On aspirin therapy at presentation
- Positive cardiac enzymes
  ● If score is 1–2, continue on heparin and check serial cardiac enzymes.
  ● If score is 3–4, consider proceed to cardiac catheterization.
  ● If score >4, start a GP IIb/IIIa inhibitor and refer for cardiac catheterization.
Also refer for cardiac catheterization if angina or ECG changes persist despite therapy or serial cardiac enzymes become elevated.

After initial therapy
Check fasting lipid and glycemic status.
Initiate and titrate statin therapy early with the goal to reduce low-density lipoprotein to less than 70 mg/dL.
Obtain an echocardiogram to assess for wall motion abnormalities and left ventricular ejection fraction.
Consider institution of an angiotensin-converting enzyme inhibitor (e.g., lisinopril, enalapril) if the patient has hypertension, diabetes, depressed left ventricular function, or presents with heart failure.

Before discharge
If a conservative strategy was employed in management (TIMI score 1–2), a low-level stress test should be performed before discharge.
  ● If high-risk result, refer for cardiac catheterization.
Educate on cardiac risk factor reduction strategies.
  ● Smoking cessation
  ● Weight loss
  ● Low fat diet
  ● Diabetes control
  ● Exercise
  ● Hypertension control

S **What are the patient's symptoms?**
The majority of patients present with severe substernal chest pain.
- May radiate to the left arm, neck, or jaw.
- Commonly associated with nausea, vomiting, dyspnea, and/or diaphoresis.

Less commonly patients may present with:
- Atypical symptoms (e.g., dyspnea alone, epigastric pain).
  - Women and diabetics tend to present with atypical symptoms.
- Heart failure (usually in the case of an extensive myocardial infarction [MI]).
- Tachyarrhythmias (e.g., ventricular tachycardia [VT]).
- Bradyarrhythmias or heart block—more common with inferior MIs.
- Cardiogenic shock or sudden cardiac death.

How long have the symptoms been present?
Ideally, revascularization therapy should be performed within 6 hours of onset of MI.

Does the patient have risk factors for cardiac disease?
- Diabetes   - Hypertension
- Tobacco abuse   - Dyslipidemia
- Family history of premature cardiac disease (less than age 55 in men; less than age 60 in women).

Inquire about cocaine use in young patients or those without other risk factors.

Does the patient have a history of coronary artery disease?

Perform a review of systems
May suggest alternative diagnoses (e.g., pericarditis, myocarditis, aortic dissection).
Inquire about bleeding abnormalities.

O **Check vital signs**
Hypotension and low oxygen saturations may indicate the onset of cardiogenic shock.
Hypertension and tachycardia can exacerbate ischemia.

Perform a directed physical examination looking for the following features
An elevated jugular venous pressure reflects increased cardiac filling pressure and suggests a right ventricular infarction if the patient is presenting with an inferior MI.
The presence of an S_3 or S_4 usually reflects ischemia.
A new mitral regurgitation murmur may indicate papillary muscle ischemia/infarction.
Congestive heart failure—may reflect diastolic dysfunction from ischemia or left ventricular systolic dysfunction from infarction or preexisting cardiomyopathy.

Obtain an electrocardiogram
ST elevation of 1 mm or more in the limb leads or 2 mm or more in the precordial leads is significant.
The leads in which ST elevation (STE) occurs indicates the affected region of the heart and the likely coronary artery involved.
- Leads V_1–V_5: anterior wall MI; left anterior descending coronary artery.
- Leads V_5–V_6, I, aVL: lateral wall MI; left circumflex artery involvement.
- Leads II, III, aVF: inferior MI; right coronary artery involvement.

A new left bundle branch block may also reflect an acute MI.
Look for evidence of heart block.

Obtain a chest x-ray
Look for signs of pulmonary edema.

Review laboratory tests
Cardiac enzymes (may be normal within the first 4–6 hours after a STEMI).
Hematocrit (consider transfusion if the hematocrit is less than 30).
Electrolytes (keep potassium greater than 4 and magnesium greater than 2 to reduce arrhythmias).

A

ST elevation myocardial infarction

Usually reflects rupture of an atherosclerotic plaque with complete thrombosis of the affected coronary artery and subsequent myocardial infarction.

Rarely the etiology may be secondary to
Coronary emboli (from valvular vegetation or intracardiac thrombi)
Vasculitis (e.g., Takayasu's arteritis, Kawasaki's disease)
Coronary artery dissection

Differential diagnosis
- Myocarditis   - Pericarditis   - Aortic dissection
- Unstable angina   - NSTEMI   - Pulmonary embolism

P

A STEMI is a medical emergency and requires prompt assessment and treatment.

Immediately start medical therapy
Aspirin 325 mg orally.
Nitroglycerin sublingually or as an IV drip as required for symptom control.
Morphine for pain control and to decrease sympathetic tone.
Intravenous metoprolol (5 mg every 5 minutes three times) followed by oral dosing (25–50 mg bid).
Start angiotensin-converting enzyme inhibitor (ACE-I) within the first 24 hours unless contraindicated.
  • Captopril 6.25 mg tid and titrate as blood pressure tolerates.
Start intravenous heparin.

Institute reperfusion therapy
Emergent catheterization and percutaneous revascularization is preferred treatment.
If cardiac catheterization cannot be performed within 3 hours, then thrombolytic agents such as tissue plasminogen activator, recombinant plasminogen activator, or tenecteplase should be administered immediately.

Admit to the coronary care unit and monitor for at least 24 hours
Check serial cardiac enzymes (every 8 hours for 24 hours) and daily electrocardiogram.
Check fasting lipids, serum glucose, and hemoglobin A1c.
  • Titrate statin therapy pending lipid results—goal low-density lipoprotein is less than 70 mg/dL.
Titrate beta-blocker and ACE-I as heart rate (HR) and blood pressure tolerate.
  • Ideal HR: ~60 beats per minute; ideal systolic blood pressure: less than 120 mm Hg.
Limit mobility in the first 48 hours. Gradually ambulate over the next 48–72 hours.

Obtain an echocardiogram to assess left ventricular function
Consider anticoagulation for 3 months if the anterior wall or left ventricular apex is akinetic.

Consider addition of eplerenone (aldosterone receptor blocker) if the patient has congestive heart failure

Aggressively treat modifiable risk factors

Consider further diagnostic testing of patients after successful thrombolytic therapy
Low level stress testing for risk stratification (72 hours after MI) *OR*
Cardiac catheterization and revascularization if significant residual coronary artery disease.

Enroll in a cardiac rehab program
Cardiac rehabilitation referral to improve patient's exercise tolerance and facilitate aggressive risk factor modification.

S

What are the patient's symptoms?

Common symptoms that may require further cardiac stress testing include:

- Exertional chest discomfort
- Dyspnea on exertion
- Symptoms similar to a previous cardiac event
- Exertional palpitations

Symptoms that likely do not require further testing include:

- Fleeting chest pain (lasts seconds at a time) or pain that is reproducible by palpation.
- Shortness of breath that is known to be noncardiac in origin.
- Asymptomatic patients.

What is the patient's pretest likelihood of coronary artery disease?

This is estimated from the patient's cardiac risk factors, including:

- Hypertension
- Diabetes mellitus
- Dyslipidemia
- Previous history of coronary artery disease (CAD)
- Tobacco use
- Obesity
- Age (male older than 45 years, female older than 55 years)
- Family history of premature CAD

The more numerous the risk factors the higher the pre-test likelihood of disease.

Can the patient exercise to a reasonable level?

A patient needs to exercise to 85% of their maximum predicted heart rate to consider the test as diagnostic (maximal predicted heart rate = 220 − (patient's age)).

Claudication, orthopedic conditions, neurologic conditions, and lung disease may limit the patient's ability to perform an exercise stress test.

Does the patient have a history of lung disease?

Asthma or severe chronic obstructive pulmonary disease are contraindications to the use of adenosine or dipyridamole during pharmacological stress testing.

Obtain a list of medications

Digoxin can cause rate related ST changes on an electrocardiogram (ECG), leading to a false positive test result.

Medications that blunt the heart rate (e.g., beta-blockers, calcium channel blockers) limit maximal heart rate during exercise and decrease the sensitivity of the stress test.

- These agents should be held for 12 hours before the test in patients in whom the test is being performed to evaluate for CAD.

O

Review vital signs

Exercise testing should not be performed if the resting blood pressure is greater than 180/100 mm Hg.

Perform a focused physical examination

Cardiac: Assess for signs of significant aortic stenosis or decompensated congestive heart failure.

- Stress testing is contraindicated in these conditions.

Pulmonary: Listen for evidence of bronchospasm (precludes use of adenosine).

Look for mechanical or neurologic limitations to exercise.

Obtain an electrocardiogram

Exclude acute ischemia or arrhythmia with a rapid ventricular response.

Look for left bundle branch block (LBBB), left ventricular hypertrophy (LVH) with strain pattern, paced rhythms, old myocardial infarction (MI) (deep Q waves).

- The ST segments may not be interpretable during stress testing.

Review laboratory studies

Exclude acute MI before stress testing in patients with a suggestive history.

Cardiac stress testing
A noninvasive test designed to identify significant CAD by increasing the heart's oxygen demand and inducing cardiac ischemia in patients with flow-limiting coronary stenoses.

Mode of stress
Exercise: The most physiologic stress; preferred in most patients who can exercise.
- Several exercise protocols exist; the Bruce protocol is used most frequently.

Pharmacologic:
- Dobutamine
  - Increases in heart rate and contractility and induces ischemia that can be seen as a new wall motion abnormality on echocardiogram.
  - May precipitate tachyarrhythmias.
- Adenosine or dipyridamole
  - Dilates normal (but not diseased) coronary arteries and induces a flow mismatch that can be seen on nuclear imaging. Rarely causes ischemia.
  - May cause bronchospasm, headaches, and chest pain.

Mode of imaging
Electrocardiogram
- Ischemia appears as ST segment depressions induced during exercise.

Nuclear scanning with technetium 99 (Myoview or MIBI) or thallium.
- The isotope is distributed in the heart in proportion to regional blood flow.
- Ischemia appears as normal myocardial perfusion at rest and decreased myocardial perfusion with stress.

Echocardiography
- Ischemia appears as an area of the left ventricle that does not contract as well after exercise as it does at rest.

Determine the appropriate stress test to perform
Can the patient walk?
- If "Yes": perform an exercise stress test.
- If "No": perform a pharmacologic stress test.

Is the ECG interpretable with exercise?
- If "Yes": ECG monitoring may be adequate.
- If "No": will need nuclear or echocardiographic imaging during the test.
  - LBBB, LVH with strain, paced rhythm, digoxin effect.

Consider an imaging study in patients with prior coronary revascularization

Consider an adenosine nuclear study in all patients with left bundle branch block

Consider an imaging modality (echocardiogram) in all women with an appropriate history

If the stress test result is positive for ischemia
Start aspirin; consider beta-blocker or calcium channel blocker to limit heart rate. Aggressive risk factor reduction.

Consider referral for cardiac catheterization if the following occur during the test
ST segment depression in greater than 5 leads.
ST segment depression greater than 2 mm or any ST elevation.
Exercise-induced decrease in systolic blood pressure (>20 mm Hg).
Chest pain or ECG changes at a low workload (less than 3 minutes of exercise or 5 METS workload).

S **What were the patient's presenting symptoms?**
- Dyspnea   - Orthopnea   - Paroxysmal nocturnal dyspnea
- Chest pain/tightness   - Palpitations   - Lower extremity edema

What is the time course of the illness?
Insidious onset of symptoms suggests gradual accumulation of fluid.
Sudden onset suggests ischemia, hypertension, or valvular disease.
A preceding viral syndrome may suggest viral myocarditis.

How limited is the patient by the symptoms?
Can be classified by the New York Heart Association (NYHA) system:
- Class I: symptoms only at significant exertion.
- Class II: symptoms with usual exertion.
- Class III: symptoms with less than usual exertion.
- Class IV: symptoms with any exertion or at rest.

Does the patient have a preexisting condition that may predispose to the development of left ventricular dysfunction?
- Coronary artery disease   - Hypertension   - Alcoholism
- Prior rheumatic fever   - Prior endocarditis   - Cocaine use

O **Review vital signs**
Patients with systolic heart failure are often tachycardic, relatively hypotensive with a narrowed pulse pressure, and with low O_2 saturation.

Perform a thorough physical examination
May appear diaphoretic, dyspneic, and in respiratory distress.
Look for evidence of volume overload:
- Pulmonary rales   - Pleural effusion   - Elevated jugular venous
- Hepatojugular reflux   - Peripheral edema   pressure
                                                 - Ascites
Look for evidence of poor perfusion:
- Cool, clammy, or mottled extremities
- Confusion
Listen for murmurs of valvular stenosis or regurgitation.
Listen for an S_3 (reflects poor left ventricular [LV] systolic function) or S_4 (indicates a stiff LV).

Review laboratories
Hyponatremia, increased blood urea nitrogen/creatinine, increased brain natriuretic peptide.

Obtain an electrocardiogram, looking for
Evidence of ischemia/infarct, tachyarrhythmia, left ventricular hypertrophy.
Left bundle branch block (LBBB):
- Patients with LBBB, low LV ejection fraction and NYHA class III–IV congestive heart failure may benefit from resynchronization therapy (see subsequent discussion).

Review the chest x-ray, looking for
- Large cardiac silhouette   - Pulmonary edema or pleural effusions

Obtain an echocardiogram
Quantify the severity of LV dysfunction and associated right ventricular (RV) dysfunction.
Assess for evidence of prior myocardial infarction.
Identify valvular disease.
Estimate right atrial, pulmonary arterial, pulmonary capillary wedge pressures.

Systolic heart failure
Weakening of the LV, leading to decreased perfusion of vital organs and both systemic and pulmonary congestion.

Differential diagnosis
 - Diastolic heart failure   - Volume overload   - Nephrotic syndrome

Stabilize acutely ill patients
Administer supplemental oxygen.
Give IV diuretics (e.g., furosemide 20–100 mg) to congested patients.
 • Follow daily weight and fluid balance closely.
 • If refractory to diuretics, consider use of nesiritide.
Give IV morphine as needed.
 • Acts as a venodilator and anxiolytic; blunts the sensation of dyspnea.

Administer intravenous medications to patients with decompensated congestive heart failure
Start dopamine in hypotensive patients.
Consider addition of inotropic agent in patients with signs of poor perfusion.
 • Dopamine, dobutamine, or milrinone.
Consider use of IV nitroglycerin or nitroprusside in hypertensive patients.

Consider use of a pulmonary arterial catheter to guide management
If the patient's volume status is unclear.
In patients with progressive renal insufficiency despite volume overload.

Begin chronic medical therapy with oral agents
Maximize afterload reduction.
 • Initiate an oral angiotensin-converting enzyme inhibitor (ACE-I) if not hypotensive (e.g., captopril 6.25 mg tid).
   ◆ Titrate to highest dose tolerated.
 • Use combination hydralazine/nitrates for ACE-I–intolerant patients.
   ◆ Consider adding to ACE-I in African American patients.
Start beta-blocker therapy when no longer volume overloaded.
 • Carvedilol 3.125 mg bid or metoprolol XL 25 mg qd initially.
Add spironolactone 25 mg qd in patients with Class III–IV symptoms.
Consider adding digoxin to ACE-I/beta-blocker if symptoms persist.

Consider biventricular pacing (resynchronization therapy)
In patients with left ventricular ejection fraction less than 35%, a wide QRS complex (>140 msec), and persistent symptoms on optimal medical therapy.

Consider implantable cardioverter/defibrillator in all patients with congestive heart failure and left ventricular ejection fraction less than 35%

Advise patient on lifestyle changes
Low salt diet (<2 g/day); consider fluid restriction to ~1.5 L/day.
Encourage exercise; consider enrollment in cardiac rehab program.

Determine etiology of left ventricular dysfunction
Perform noninvasive testing or cardiac catheterization to exclude coronary artery disease.
Check thyroid function tests, iron studies.
Consider right ventricle endomyocardial biopsy if infiltrative disease suspected.

S **What are the patient's symptoms?**

May be impossible to differentiate from those of systolic heart failure (see SOAP 13).

- Dyspnea on exertion   • Orthopnea   • Paroxysmal nocturnal dyspnea
- Lower extremity edema   • Fatigue   • Chest pain/tightness

Obtain a medical history

Hypertension is the most common cause of diastolic heart failure (DHF).

Ischemia can predispose to both systolic and DHF.

- Diastole is more energy dependent and more affected by ischemia.

Infiltrative disorders including hemochromatosis, amyloidosis, and sarcoidosis.

Aortic stenosis, even when mild in severity, can cause diastolic heart failure.

Is the patient compliant with medications and dietary restrictions?

Patients with hypertension often present with DHF during periods of noncompliance.

 Review vital signs

Tachycardia, especially atrial fibrillation (AF), is poorly tolerated in DHF.

- Tachycardia shortens diastole and thereby limits diastolic filling.
- Loss of atrial contraction in AF significantly reduces ventricular filling.

Perform a cardiac examination

An S_4 gallop is almost always present in DHF.

A systolic ejection murmur is often heard.

- May reflect a dynamic mid-left ventricular (LV) cavity gradient or LV outflow tract gradient in patients with severe left ventricular hypertrophy (LVH) or hypertrophic cardiomyopathy.

A loud P_2 will be present in patients with chronic DHF and pulmonary HTN.

Perform a directed extracardiac examination looking for

Hypertensive retinopathy.

Evidence of pulmonary congestion.

Evidence of volume overload (increased jugular venous pressure, edema).

Vascular bruits.

- Abdominal bruits may indicate renal artery stenosis as a cause of DHF.

Obtain an electrocardiogram

Assess for acute or chronic ischemic changes, LVH, left atrial enlargement.

Review the chest x-ray

Assess cardiac size and presence of pulmonary edema.

Exclude obvious pulmonary cause of dyspnea (e.g., chronic obstructive pulmonary disease, infection, tumor).

Review laboratory data

Renal impairment predisposes to volume overload and may aggravate diastolic heart failure.

Plasma levels of brain natriuretic peptide (BNP) are usually elevated.

- BNP cannot differentiate systolic from diastolic dysfunction.

Request an echocardiogram

Patients with DHF have normal or supra-normal LV systolic function.

Diastolic dysfunction can be graded (I–IV) using tissue Doppler techniques.

- Assesses diastolic relaxation of the LV.
- Can estimate ventricular filling pressure.

A

Diastolic heart failure
Cardiac dysfunction in which left ventricular *filling* is abnormal and is accompanied by elevated filling pressures. Systolic function (LV ejection fraction) is preserved and significant valvular disease is absent.

Common etiologies
- Hypertension
- Myocardial ischemia
- Pericardial constriction (See SOAP 21)
- Hypertrophic cardiomyopathy
- Infiltrative disorders

Differential diagnosis
- Systolic heart failure
- "High output" heart failure
- Lung disease
- Valvular heart disease
- Renal artery stenosis
- Inadequate dialysis in end-stage renal disease

P

Admit patients with decompensated diastolic heart failure

Administer supplemental oxygen by nasal cannula or face mask

Administer diuretics as needed to control congestive symptoms
Loop diuretics are preferred (e.g., furosemide).
Need to avoid overdiuresis as volume depletion will worsen diastolic dysfunction and may induce hypotension.
Follow daily weights and fluid balance closely.

Control heart rate
Beta-blockers and calcium channel blockers are preferred.
- Aim for a goal heart rate of ~50–60 beats per minute.
- A slower HR provides more time for diastolic filling of the LV.
- The negatively inotropic effects of these medications may improve LV relaxation.

Control hypertension
If severe (systolic blood pressure >180 mm Hg) in face of acute DHF, consider use of intravenous nitroprusside or enalaprilat.
Beta-blockers, calcium channel blockers, angiotensin-converting enzyme inhibitors, and angiotensin receptor blockers have theoretical benefits over other agents for chronic management.
- May improve diastolic function.

Consider performing cardioversion in patients with atrial fibrillation or flutter
Loss of atrial contraction significantly worsens diastolic function.

Place on a low sodium diet (<2 g Na⁺/day)

Evaluate for ischemia in patients who do not have an obvious cause for diastolic heart failure
Coronary revascularization should be performed if ischemia is thought to be contributing to DHF.

S **What are the patient's symptoms?**
Common presenting symptoms of right heart failure (RHF) include:
- Fatigue
- Lethargy
- Dyspnea
- Decreased appetite
- Lower extremity edema
- Increasing abdominal girth

Obtain a medical history
Left-sided heart failure.
- The most common cause of RHF is left heart failure.

Coronary artery disease.
- Inferior MI is frequently associated with right ventricular infarction and RHF.

Severe or long-standing lung disease.
- RHF secondary to lung disease is referred to as cor pulmonale.

Congenital heart disease.
- Intracardiac shunts (i.e., atrial or ventricular septal defect).
- Pulmonary stenosis.

Tricuspid valve disease (e.g., endocarditis, carcinoid, Epstein's anomaly).
Liver cirrhosis, nephrotic syndrome, and causes of low serum protein can lead to signs and symptoms similar to those of right heart failure.

Perform a thorough review of systems
The presence of orthopnea or paroxysmal nocturnal dyspnea in addition to the symptoms of RHF suggests associated left heart failure.

O **Review vital signs**

Perform a physical examination looking for
Elevated jugular venous pressure.
A right ventricular S_3 and a right-ventricular heave.
A loud pulmonary component of the second heart sound.
- Suggests the presence of pulmonary hypertension.

A murmur of tricuspid regurgitation.
Pulsatile hepatomegaly (indicates tricuspid regurgitation) and ascites.
Bilateral lower extremity pitting edema.

Perform electrocardiography
Look for evidence of right atrial enlargement (P wave >2.5 mm tall in lead II).
Look for evidence of right ventricular hypertrophy.
- RsR' pattern in lead V_1
- R wave >7 mm tall in lead V_1
- Right axis deviation
- S wave > R wave in lead V_6

Perform chest radiography
Evaluate for evidence of chronic lung disease or pulmonary edema.
Look for evidence of pulmonary hypertension and RV enlargement.

Review laboratory tests
Anemia may aggravate heart failure symptoms.
Check renal and hepatic function, albumin, thyroid-stimulating hormone.
- Cirrhosis, nephrotic syndrome, hypoalbuminemia, and hypothyroidism can cause edema, ascites, and fatigue, and mimic the signs and symptoms of RHF.

A **Right heart failure**
Inability of the right ventricle to maintain an adequate cardiac output resulting in signs and symptoms of systemic venous congestion and/or organ hypoperfusion.

Etiology
RV pressure overload
 • Pulmonary hypertension (primary or secondary), pulmonary stenosis
RV volume overload
 • Atrial or ventricular septal defects, tricuspid regurgitation
Disorders affecting the RV myocardium
 • RV infarction (usually in association with an inferior MI)
 • Myocarditis
 • Infiltrative disorders (e.g., amyloidosis)

Differential diagnosis
 - Cirrhosis   - Nephrotic syndrome   - Hypothyroidism
 - Pericardial constriction   - Volume overload states

P **Stabilize patients with acute RHF**
Hemodynamically unstable patients require inotropic support (e.g., dopamine, dobutamine), and volume resuscitation (even if volume overloaded).
Patients with RHF that is refractory to inotropic therapy may require a right ventricular assist device for stabilization and as a bridge to cardiac transplant.

Begin diuretic therapy when patients are stable and in patients with chronic RHF
Oral loop diuretics (e.g., furosemide) to control systemic venous congestion.
 • Administer intravenously in the acute setting.
Consider addition of spironolactone in patients with ascites.
 • May require intermittent paracentesis.

Obtain an echocardiogram
Assess the size and function of the right ventricle.
Estimate pulmonary pressures.
Exclude left-sided heart failure and mitral or aortic valve disease.
Evaluate for atrial septal defect (ASD) or ventricular septal defect (VSD) with color Doppler techniques and with injection of agitated saline ("bubble study").
Assess for tricuspid regurgitation and pulmonary valvular stenosis.
Exclude pericardial disease.

Consider cardiac catheterization
 - Confirm pulmonary hypertension   - Assess for coronary artery disease

Consider performing pulmonary function testing and ventilation-perfusion scan
If pulmonary disease is the suspected cause.

Treat reversible causes of RHF
Treat left heart failure with usual medications. (See SOAP 11.)
Epoprostenol infusion for primary pulmonary hypertension. (See SOAP 54.)
Consider closure of ASD or VSD.
Consider surgical correction of valvular disease.

Encourage moderate sodium (<2 g/day) and water restriction (~1.5 L/day)

S

What are the patient's symptoms?
Up to 90% of patients with hypertrophic cardiomyopathy (HCM) are asymptomatic at the time of initial diagnosis.

When present, common presenting symptoms include:
- Dyspnea on exertion
- Postural lightheadedness
- Fatigue
- Chest pain
- Palpitations
- Edema
- Presyncope or syncope
- Sudden death

Obtain a medical history
Investigate for other potential causes of cardiac hypertrophy/thickening including:
- Severe hypertension
- Valvular heart disease
- Infiltrative cardiac disorders (e.g., amyloidosis)

Obtain a family history
Ask about a family history of HCM or of sudden cardiac death.

Perform a thorough review of systems
Syncope or presyncope is associated with an increased mortality rate.

O

Review vital signs
Uncontrolled hypertension can cause left ventricular hypertrophy (LVH) and mimic HCM.

Perform a cardiac examination looking for
Hyperdynamic left ventricular apical impulse. An apical systolic thrill may be present.

Harsh, crescendo-decrescendo systolic murmur heard best at the left sternal border. Several features differentiate the murmur of HCM from mitral regurgitation or aortic stenosis:

- The murmur of HCM is the only left-sided murmur that becomes louder during expiration and with sustained Valsalva maneuver.
- The murmur may be decreased by sitting or squatting, with handgrip, or following passive elevation of the legs.
- The carotid pulse is brisk and bifid in nature (as opposed to the slow rising and diminished nature of the pulse in aortic stenosis).

A prominent S_4 is common.

Obtain an electrocardiograph (ECG); characteristic findings include
LVH: the QRS voltage increases with increasing LV hypertrophy.

Left axis deviation and left atrial enlargement.

Prominent deep Q waves may be seen in the inferior and lateral leads.
- Reflect septal depolarization of the hypertrophied tissue.

Obtain an echocardiogram; characteristic features include
Marked left (and often right) ventricular hypertrophy (often >15 mm).
- LVH may be concentric, apical, or asymmetric.

A dynamic gradient in the mid LV cavity or the LV outflow tract (LVOT).

Systolic anterior motion (SAM) of the mitral valve +/− mitral regurgitation.
- The mitral apparatus is pulled into the LV outflow tract by the accelerated flow across the dynamic gradient.

Evidence of diastolic dysfunction.

LV dilation and systolic dysfunction develop in 10% to 15% of patients with HCM.

A **Hypertrophic cardiomyopathy**
An autosomal dominant condition with variable penetrance that causes myocyte hypertrophy and disarray and produces a phenotypic appearance that varies from normal to marked asymmetric LV hypertrophy.

Differential diagnosis
-Hypertensive heart disease   - Aortic stenosis
- Storage disorders (e.g., Fabry's disease)
- Infiltrative disorders (e.g., amyloidosis, hemochromatosis)

Prognosis
The risk of sudden cardiac death (SCD) is 1% to 6% per year.
High-risk features include:
- LVOT gradient >20 mm Hg
- Age <45 years
- Family history of sudden death
- History of syncope or SCD

P **Consider further testing if diagnosis is unclear by echocardiography**
Magnetic resonance imaging is particularly useful if echo images are poor quality.
May also be superior to echo for identification of isolated apical hypertrophy.
Endomyocardial biopsy will demonstrate characteristic abnormalities.
- Performed via a bioptome introduced through the jugular vein.
Genetic testing: Many genetic mutations have now been identified. Certain mutations portend a worse prognosis and require more aggressive treatment.

Initiate medical therapy in symptomatic patients
Beta-blockers and calcium channel blockers (often at high dose).
- Slow the heart rate and thereby improve LV diastolic filling.
- The negative inotropic effects may reduce the dynamic gradient.
Disopyramide (has negative inotropic effects) may also be effective.
Congestive symptoms are treated with loop diuretics.
- Use with caution as volume depletion will induce hypotension.

Consider septal ablation if symptoms persist despite optimal medical therapy
Consider in patient with severe LVOT gradient (>50 mm Hg).
Reduces LVOT gradient; improves symptoms in 90% of patients.
May be performed surgically or by the percutaneous infusion of alcohol into the septal coronary arterial branches.

Perform noninvasive testing of asymptomatic patients to identify high-risk markers
Stress testing: Evaluate for exertional hypotension/presyncope/syncope.
Ambulatory ECG monitoring: Evaluate for ventricular arrhythmias.
Unclear if empiric medical therapy is indicated in low-risk patients.

Consider electrophysiologic device therapy
An implantable cardioverter-defibrillator should be placed in patients with high-risk of SCD.
The role of dual chamber pacing is uncertain.

Screen all first degree family members of patients with HCM
Perform a thorough screening history, physical examination, ECG, and echocardiogram, even if they are asymptomatic.

S **What are the patient's symptoms?**

Most patients present with signs and symptoms of heart failure, including:
- Dyspnea and fatigue
- Orthopnea
- Lower extremity edema
- Cough when lying flat
- Paroxysmal nocturnal dyspnea
- Decreased appetite

Occasionally patients remain asymptomatic and the diagnosis is made incidentally after an abnormal electrocardiograph (ECG), chest radiograph, or echocardiogram is discovered.

Does the patient have risk factors for developing a dilated cardiomyopathy (DCM)?

- Coronary artery disease
- Previous myocarditis
- Valvular heart disease
- Connective tissue disorder
- Previous myocardial infarction (MI)
- Alcoholism
- Congenital heart disease
- Persistent tachycardia
- Hypertension
- Recent pregnancy
- Cocaine abuse
- Hypothyroidism

Perform a thorough review of systems

Is there a family history of DCM?

As many as 20% of cases of DCM may be familial.

O **Check vital signs**

Tachycardia and hypotension are frequently present, especially if the patient presents in decompensated heart failure.

A narrow pulse pressure is a sign of low cardiac output.

Perform a physical examination

Dyspnea at rest and an inability to lie flat suggest decompensated congestive heart failure (CHF).

Estimate jugular venous pressure.

Cardiac: Listen carefully for both stenotic and regurgitant valve disease as both can precipitate left ventricular (LV) failure. Listen also for an S_3 or S_4.

Pulmonary: Listen for crackles and assess for pleural effusions.

Abdomen: check for hepatomegaly and ascites.

Lower extremities: check for bilateral pitting edema.

Obtain an electrocardiograph

DCM is often associated with bundle branch block, interventricular conduction delay, and left axis deviation on ECG.

Look for changes of active or previous ischemia, changes secondary to hypertension (left ventricular hypertrophy with strain), and also for evidence of tachyarrhythmias.

Obtain a chest radiograph

Signs of CHF include pulmonary edema, pleural effusions, and cardiomegaly.

Exclude overt pulmonary causes of dyspnea (infection, neoplasia, chronic obstructive pulmonary disease, etc).

Request a complete blood cell count and electrolytes

Significant anemia can cause high output failure.

Confirm renal function and electrolyte levels prior to initiating therapy.

Consider obtaining a brain natriuretic peptide level

Can be used to help determine the patient's volume status.

Is elevated in patients with decompensated CHF (normal level: <100 pg/mL).

The brain natriuretic peptide level when the patient is euvolemic can be used later as a baseline to determine if further diuresis or titration of medications is required.

A **Dilated cardiomyopathy**
The end result of a variety of conditions that result in a dilated LV with depressed systolic function. Often associated with dilation of the right ventricle and the atria.

Functional assessment and prognosis
The New York Heart Association (NYHA) classification is used to assess functional capacity and has been shown to accurately predict prognosis:
- NYHA class I: No symptoms with usual activity; <10% 1-year mortality.
- NYHA class II: Symptoms with usual activity.
- NYHA class III: Symptoms with less than usual activity.
- NYHA class IV: Symptoms with minimal physical activity or at rest; 1 yr mortality as high as 50%.

Etiology (see risk factors in previous "S" section)

P **Admit the patient**
If symptomatic with chest pain, tachycardia, or heart failure.

Obtain an echocardiogram (if not performed in the recent past)
Diagnostic modality of choice in DCM.
Can reveal the extent of cardiac chamber dilation, quantify LV function, and assess for evidence of ischemia or valvular heart disease.

Check thyroid function tests and iron level in all patients with new DCM

Obtain an exercise test or cardiac catheterization in patients with suspected coronary artery disease

Treat the underlying etiology of LV dysfunction
Coronary revascularization if etiology is ischemic.
Immediate cessation of alcohol and other substance abuse.
Avoid future pregnancy in postpartum cardiomyopathy.
Thyroid replacement in patients with hypothyroidism.
Control of hypertension and tachyarrhythmias.

Institute medical therapy to control symptoms and reduce mortality
Start angiotensin-converting enzyme inhibitor (ACEI) and titrate to the highest dose tolerated (e.g., captopril 50 mg tid, lisinopril 40 mg qd).
Start beta-blockers at low dose and slowly titrate over several weeks (e.g., start carvedilol 3.125 bid or Toprol XL 25 mg qd).
Use loop diuretics (e.g., furosemide) to control congestive symptoms.
Use hydralazine (25 to 100 mg tid) and nitrates (120 mg qd) as alternative or additive therapy to ACEI inhibitors.
Consider adding digoxin (0.125 mg qd) in patients with persistent symptoms.
Add spironolactone for survival benefit in patients with class III or IV CHF.

Counsel patient regarding dietary changes
2 g/day sodium diet and a 1.5 L fluid restriction.
Weight should be followed daily.

Consider resynchronization therapy (biventricular pacing) for qualifying patients
NYHA class III/VI CHF, left ventricular ejection fraction <30%, QRS duration >160 msec on ECG.

Consider placement of an implantable cardiac defibrillator in patients with a left ventricular ejection fraction of <35%
Provides mortality benefit in patients with ischemic or nonischemic cardiomyopathy, regardless of whether there has been a documented ventricular arrhythmia.

S **What were the patient's presenting symptoms?**
Many patients with myocarditis are asymptomatic.
Symptomatic patients may present with:
- Chest pain (often pleuritic)
- Viral syndrome (fevers, chills, myalgias, fatigue)
- Congestive heart failure, hemodynamic instability
- Tachycardia, palpitations, syncope, sudden cardiac death

Obtain a thorough medical history
A history of an antecedent viral illness is often present.
Inquire about noninfectious factors that may predispose to myocarditis:
- Chemotherapeutic agents (e.g., anthracyclines, fluorouracil).
- History of connective tissue disorders – rheumatoid arthritis, sarcoidosis.
- Substance abuse (e.g., cocaine, alcohol).
- Other toxic exposures including arsenic, lead, snake bite, tick bites.

Does the patient have risk factors for coronary artery disease?
Symptoms of myocarditis can mimic those of ischemia; the absence of cardiac risk factors makes ischemia less likely.

 Obtain a travel history
Lyme disease is endemic in New England and California.
Chagas disease is endemic in parts of rural South America.

Obtain vital signs
Most symptomatic patients are tachycardic, tachypneic, and often hypoxic.
Signs of shock (hypotension and organ hypoperfusion) may be present in patients with fulminant myocarditis.

Search for extra cardiac manifestations of illnesses that cause myocarditis
Rashes (e.g., erythema nodosum in sarcoidosis, malar rash of systemic lupus erythematosus [SLE], target lesion of Lyme disease).
Lymphadenopathy (may suggest sarcoidosis).

Perform a cardiac examination, looking specifically for
Signs of heart failure (elevated jugular venous pressure, a third or fourth heart sound).
The murmur of mitral or tricuspid regurgitation may be present.
A pericardial friction rub is often present and reflects concomitant pericarditis.

Obtain an electrocardiograph
Common findings include: sinus tachycardia, diffuse T wave inversions.
Heart block or transient ST elevation may be seen.
Evidence of associated pericarditis is often present. (See SOAP 18.)

Review laboratory studies
Chest radiograph often reveals an enlarged cardiac silhouette and pulmonary edema.
Leukocytosis is common.
Erythrocyte sedimentation rate (ESR) is usually elevated (often >100).
Creatine kinase and troponin are elevated in the acute phase of myocarditis.
- May remain elevated for several days, as opposed to myocardial infarction in which the enzymes usually peak within 12 to 24 hours.

Myocarditis
An inflammatory disease of the myocardium resulting in systolic dysfunction.
Diagnosis suspected on clinical grounds; can only be confirmed by right ventricular
biopsy.

Etiology
Infectious. Most common organisms include:
- Viral: coxsackie, adenovirus, enterovirus, HIV.
- Bacterial: tuberculosis, diphtheria, brucellosis.
- Fungal: candida, histoplasma.
- Protozoal: trypanosoma cruzi (Chagas disease)
- Rickettsial: typhus, Q fever.
- Spirochetal: borrelia (Lyme disease).
Systemic disease (e.g., sarcoid, rheumatoid arthritis, SLE, rheumatic fever).
Toxic/drug induced (e.g., cocaine, catecholamines, anthracyclines, alcohol).
Hypersensitivity reactions (e.g., antibiotics, insect stings, snake bites).

Differential diagnosis
Myocardial ischemia/infarction: tends to be acute in onset, associated with evolu-
tionary ECG changes and transient increase in cardiac enzymes.
- May require coronary angiography to differentiate from myocarditis.
Pericarditis (without myocarditis): produces pleuritic chest pain with diffuse ST
elevation but no elevation in cardiac enzymes or change in left ventricle (LV) function.

**Admit patients with acute myocarditis to telemetry floor or to the cardiac
care unit**

Obtain an echocardiogram
Usually reveals global LV systolic dysfunction. Right ventricle involvement is common.
May reveal mitral regurgitation or tricuspid regurgitation, pericardial effusion,
intracardiac thrombi.

Determine specific cause of myocarditis
Consider obtaining viral, borrelia, or trypanosomal antibodies if suspected.
Consider endomyocardial biopsy if collagen vascular or infiltrative disease is sus-
pected, or in patients in whom the diagnosis of myocarditis is uncertain.

Treat the underlying cause, if identified
Antibiotics if a bacterial source of infection is identified.
Stop suspected drug or remove offending toxin.
Aggressively treat systemic or infiltrative disorders.

Institute standard medical therapy
Conventional treatment for congestive heart failure (CHF), including diuretics,
angiotensin converting enzyme inhibitors, beta-blockers (if possible), digoxin.
Anticoagulation with warfarin if left ventricle or left atria thrombi or severely
depressed left ventricular ejection fraction.
There is no benefit of routine use of immunosuppressive medications.
- May be indicated in specific cases (e.g., SLE, giant cell myocarditis).
Avoid exercise during acute phase of myocarditis; avoid alcohol and NSAIDs.

Consider more aggressive therapy for decompensated patients
Transcutaneous or transvenous pacing for heart block.
Inotropic agents and/or intraaortic balloon pump for intractable CHF.

Consider heart transplantation
In acute illness if unable to wean off mechanical support devices.
In chronic illness in a patient with recurrent decompensated CHF.

S **What are the patient's symptoms?**
Most patients with shock are systemically ill and cannot provide a history. Family
members or witnesses may give information relating to:
- Recent cardiac symptoms: chest pain, congestive heart failure (CHF) symptoms,
  palpitations, syncope.
- Cardiac history: myocardial infarction (MI), CHF, cardiomyopathy, arrhythmias,
  risk factors.

When did the patient's symptoms begin?
50% to 75% of cardiogenic shock after MI occurs within 24 hours of presentation.
Delayed shock (3 to 5 days after MI) may occur as a result of a mechanical complication of MI (papillary muscle rupture, free wall rupture, ventricular septal defect).

Are there other causes of shock to explain the patient's current state?
Sepsis: Has the patient had fevers, chills, and other infectious symptoms?
Hypovolemia: Has the patient had diarrhea, vomiting, hematemesis, bloody stool,
  melena, traumatic blood loss, or decreased oral intake?
Anaphylaxis: Ask about new medications, and prior food and drug allergies.
Pulmonary embolism: Has the patient had pleuritic chest pain? Does the patient
  have symptoms or risk factors for deep venous thrombosis?
Medications or intoxications: Has the patient been taking new or excessive anti-
  hypertensive agents? Is there reason to suspect drug abuse or toxic ingestion?
Adrenal insufficiency: Has the patient been on chronic steroid therapy?

O **Check the vital signs**
Patients are usually tachycardic, hypotensive, tachypneic, and hypoxic.
Check BP in both arms (? dissection) and check pulsus paradox (? tamponade).

Evaluate for signs of organ hypoperfusion
Assess mental status: Confusion or obtundation reflects poor cerebral perfusion.
The skin may appear pale or mottled with lacey discoloration (livedo reticularis).
The extremities are usually cool and clammy (vasoconstriction) with cardiogenic
  and hypovolemic shock, but are warm (vasodilation) with septic shock.
Oliguria (<30 cc/hr of urine output) is a sign of renal hypoperfusion.

Perform a thorough examination
Assess jugular venous pressure and listen for an S_3 or S_4, suggesting heart failure.
Listen for the murmur of mitral regurgitation, aortic stenosis or insufficiency, or
  ventricular septal defect.
Listen for a pericardial rub or muffled heart sounds (exclude pericardial effusion).
Assess the size of the abdominal aorta (exclude aneurysm).
Listen for pulmonary rales indicative of heart failure.
- The absence of CHF in cardiogenic shock suggests right ventricle (RV) infarction.
Abdomen: Exclude an acute abdominal "catastrophe" (e.g., perforated viscus).

Review the chest radiograph, looking for evidence of
- Pulmonary congestion	- Pneumothorax
- Pericardial effusion	- Pneumonia

Obtain a 12-lead electrocardiograph
Look for ST elevation or depression (ischemia/infarction), low voltage (pericardial
  effusion), or right heart strain (S1Q3T3, new right bundle branch block) suggesting
  pulmonary embolism.
If signs of acute inferior MI, obtain right-sided ECG to assess for RV infarction.

Review laboratories
Chemistries: acidosis, renal or hepatic dysfunction, elevated cardiac enzymes.
Complete blood cell count: anemia, leukocytosis.
Arterial blood gas: acidosis, hypoxemia.

Cardiogenic shock
A state of inadequate tissue perfusion resulting from reduced cardiac output. Most commonly results from an acute myocardial infarction (develops in up to 7% of MIs) where its presence indicates infarction of greater than 40% of the left ventricle. May also result from acute mitral or aortic regurgitation, acute ventricular septal defect, aortic dissection, or tamponade.

Prognosis
>60% in-hospital mortality.

 Admit to the intensive care unit

Consult cardiology

Stabilize the respiratory status
Intubation/mechanical ventilation is often required.

Stabilize blood pressure
Give empiric fluid bolus (250 cc saline) to patients without pulmonary congestion. Start dopamine for BP support and add dobutamine if suspect low cardiac output. Consider placement of an arterial catheter for continuous BP monitoring.

Consider placement of an intraaortic balloon pump if BP is not rapidly stabilized.

- Balloon inflation augments diastolic BP and coronary blood flow.
- Balloon deflation reduces afterload and improves cardiac output.

Correct acidosis and electrolyte disorders
Vasopressors are ineffective with a serum pH <7.20.

Obtain an echocardiogram (immediately)
Quantify LV and RV function and assess for mitral and aortic regurgitation, ventricular septal rupture, tamponade, and proximal aortic dissection.

Perform right heart catheterization
Hemodynamic criteria for cardiogenic shock include systemic systolic BP <90 mm Hg (or requiring pressors), pulmonary capillary wedge pressure (PCWP) >18 mm Hg, and cardiac index <2.2 L/min/m^2.
If hypovolemia or RV infarction, give IV fluids to increase pulmonary capillary wedge pressure to 16 to 18 mm Hg.
Check right atrial and pulmonary arterial O_2 saturation to exclude ventricular septal defect (VSD).
Use serial hemodynamic measurements to guide therapy.

Perform coronary angiography and revascularization in patients with acute MI
~70% of patients with cardiogenic shock have left main or 3-vessel coronary artery disease.

Percutaneous coronary intervention (PCI) of the infarct-related artery significantly reduces mortality.

- Thrombolysis is less effective but should be used if PCI is not available.
- Immediate coronary artery bypass grafting should be considered for all patients with multivessel or left main coronary artery disease.

Refer patients with cardiogenic shock from papillary muscle rupture, LV free wall rupture, acute aortic insufficiency, or acute VSD for emergent surgical repair

Assess for other causes of shock if hemodynamics or response to medications suggests an alternative diagnosis

S **What are the patient's current symptoms?**
The most prominent symptom of pericarditis is chest pain.
Constitutional symptoms are common: fevers, fatigue, and myalgias.

What is the character of the patient's chest pain?
Pericardial pain is usually sharp, substernal, moderate to severe in intensity, pleuritic (worsened on inspiration), and improved when sitting forward.
May radiate to the shoulder or scapula, and may be associated with dyspnea.

Does the patient have any condition that may predispose to pericarditis?
Myocardial infarction
- Acute myocardial infarction (MI) may be associated with regional pericarditis overlying the infarcted myocardium.
- Immune-mediated pericarditis can develop weeks to months after an acute MI (Dressler's syndrome).

Recent viral syndrome
- Coxsackie A and B, echovirus, adenovirus, Epstein-Barr virus, HIV.

Malignancy
- Most common to involve pericardium: lung, breast, lymphoma, melanoma.

Renal failure/uremia
Prior tuberculosis
Recent chest trauma or thoracic surgery
Autoimmune disease
- Systemic lupus erythematosus, rheumatoid arthritis, scleroderma.

Prior chest/mediastinal radiation

O **Review vital signs**
Tachycardia and low grade fever may be present.

The presence of tachycardia, hypotension, and elevated pulsus paradox should raise the suspicion for pericardial tamponade. (See SOAP 20.)

Perform focused physical examination looking for
Jugular venous distention: reflects elevated right atrial pressure and may indicate accumulation of pericardial fluid.

Pericardial rub is pathognomonic for pericarditis.
- Classically has 3 components reflecting atrial systole, ventricular systole, and ventricular diastole.
- A coarse, scratchy sound heard best with the diaphragm of the stethoscope and with the patient leaning forward.

Evidence of underlying disease that may cause pericarditis.

Obtain an electrocardiogram: Classic evolution of findings include
Stage 1: diffuse, concave-upward ST segment elevation; PR segment depression (usually seen best in lead II, V_5, V_6).
Stage 2: normalization of ST and PR segments.
Stage 3: diffuse T wave inversions.
Stage 4: resolution of T wave changes.
Low QRS voltage and electrical alternans may be seen if there is a large pericardial effusion.

Review laboratory data
White blood cell count is frequently elevated.
Neutropenia, thrombocytopenia may be indicative of an autoimmune process.
An elevated erythrocyte sedimentation rate indicates an inflammatory process.

Elevated cardiac enzymes (CK-MB, troponin) indicate associated myocardial injury (myocarditis or myocardial infarction).

Pericarditis
Pericarditis is an inflammatory process involving the pericardium. There may be minimal associated exudate (dry pericarditis) or there may be excessive exudate resulting in accumulation of fluid in the pericardial space (pericardial effusion).

Most common etiologies (noted previously)

Differential diagnosis
- Angina	- Pleurisy	- Myocardial infarction
- Pneumonia	- Costochondritis	- Pulmonary embolism

Features that differentiate pericarditis from MI.
Infarct pain is usually not pleuritic or positional.
ST elevation with MI is concave-downward and regional (not diffuse).
Reciprocal ST depression may be seen with MI.
PR segment depression is not present with MI.
Q waves do not develop with pericarditis.

P

Start anti-inflammatory agents in symptomatic patients
NSAIDs are the treatment of choice.
- Ibuprofen 400 to 800 mg tid, Indocin 25 to 50 mg tid, or aspirin 2 to 6 g/day.
Colchicine 0.6 mg bid may be added if NSAIDs not effective.
Steroids should be reserved only for refractory cases.

Consider obtaining an echocardiogram
Especially when concomitant myocarditis or pericardial effusion is suspected.

Obtain serial ECGs to follow evolutionary changes

Identify underlying disorders
Check antinuclear antibodies (autoimmune disease), PPD (TB), HIV (when appropriate), chest radiograph (lung cancer), breast examination (breast cancer), blood urea nitrogen/creatinine (uremia).

Treat or correct underlying disorders
Uremia: Begin or intensify dialysis.
Malignancy: Consider pericardiocentesis and send fluid for cytologic evaluation.
  Specific therapy depends on the cytology of the primary tumor.
Tuberculosis: If suspected, plant PPD, culture pericardial fluid, and consider pericardial biopsy if diagnosis still uncertain. Start antituberculous therapy (INH, rifampin, pyrazinamide, ethambutol) if TB confirmed.
Autoimmune disorders: Consider steroids.

S

How was the pericardial effusion diagnosed?
Chest radiograph: enlarged cardiac silhouette.
Echocardiogram: direct visualization of pericardial fluid.
Computed tomography (CT): direct visualization of pericardial fluid.

Does the patient have any symptoms attributable to the effusion?
Many patients will be asymptomatic and the pericardial effusion is an incidental
  finding on chest radiograph, CT scan, or echocardiogram.
Potential symptoms:
  • Pleuritic chest pain (pericarditis)
  • Dyspnea ⎫
  • Presyncope ⎬ May signify pericardial tamponade
  • Syncope ⎭

**Does the patient have any condition that is associated with pericardial
effusions?**
Any condition that causes pericarditis can cause a pericardial effusion.
  • ~60% of moderate to large effusions are the result of a known underlying
    condition.
Most common causes include:
  • Malignancy (lung, breast, lymphoma, melanoma): ~15% to 20% of cases.
  • Uremia: ~6% to 12% of cases.
  • Myocardial infarction: 8% to 10% of cases.
  • Viral/idiopathic pericarditis: 20% to 30% of cases.
Other causes include:
  • Collagen vascular disease: systemic lupus, rheumatoid arthritis.
  • Iatrogenic: following angioplasty, cardiac surgery.
  • Infectious: tuberculosis, bacterial.
  • Hypothyroidism.
  • Chest trauma.
  • Aortic dissection.
  • Medications: procainamide, hydralazine, minoxidil, isoniazid.

O

Assess vital signs
Hypotension and tachycardia may indicate progression to tamponade, a medical
  emergency. This is supported by the presence of a pulsus paradoxus. (See SOAP 20.)

Perform a physical examination
General: may appear dyspneic at rest.
Heart:
  • Elevated jugular venous pressure: indicates increased right heart pressure.
  • Diminished heart sounds: results from poor sound transmission through fluid.
  • Pericardial rub:
    ◆ If present, indicates active pericarditis.
    ◆ Often absent with large effusion because the layers of the pericardium are no
      longer in contact.
Chest:
  • Evidence of a pleural effusion (decreased breath sounds and dullness to percus-
    sion at the lung bases).
  • Left lower lobe atelectasis due to compression of the lung.
  • Dullness to percussion under the left scapula (Ewart's sign) resulting from the
    large pericardial effusion.

Review chest radiogram
Cardiomegaly with a globular cardiac silhouette ("water bottle heart").
Evidence of lung disease (effusions, infiltrates, masses).

Obtain an electrocardiogram
With large effusions may see:
- Low QRS voltage.
- Electrical alternans (alternating QRS axis); due to the heart's rhythmic motion within the pericardial fluid.

 Pericardial effusion
The visceral pericardium is adherent to the epicardium and is separated from the parietal pericardium by the pericardial space, which normally contains less than 50 cc of lubricating fluid.
Excess fluid may accumulate in the pericardial space as a result of any process that causes pericarditis.
Most common causes as outlined previously.

 Confirm presence of a pericardial effusion

If pericardial effusion is suspected on the basis of history, examination, chest radiograph, or CT scan findings, it should always be confirmed with an echocardiogram.
Echocardiography can:
- Determine size of the effusion.
- Determine hemodynamic significance of the effusion.
- Identify structural heart disease (evidence of myocardial infarction, aortic aneurysm).

Assess hemodynamic significance of effusion (see SOAP 20)
Check for hypotension, elevated JVP, increased pulsus paradox.
Admit to ICU and perform urgent pericardiocentesis in hemodynamically unstable patients.

Perform selected tests to search for possible causes
Chest radiograph (? lung cancer), blood urea nitrogen/creatinine (uremia), thyroid-stimulating hormone (hypothyroidism), erythrocyte sedimentation rate (inflammatory disease), antinuclear antigen (collagen vascular disease), HIV, PPD (TB), breast examination/mammography (? breast cancer)

Consider diagnostic pericardiocentesis if a moderate or large effusion persists (>1 week) or etiology unknown
Send fluid for cytology, bacterial culture, acid-fast bacillus stain and culture.
Fluid protein, lactate dehydrogenase, glucose, pH, cell count are of little value.
Pericardial biopsy may be helpful if previous evaluation unrevealing.

Consider obtaining a pericardial biopsy if etiology remains uncertain

Treat identified underlying cause

S **What are the patient's symptoms?**
Acute tamponade: dyspnea, lightheadedness, presyncope, or syncope.
  • May present with hemodynamic collapse.
Subacute tamponade: dyspnea, fatigue, pedal edema.

Does the patient have any conditions that predispose to pericardial effusions/tamponade?
Any condition that causes a pericardial effusion can cause pericardial tamponade. (See SOAP 19.)
Most common causes of pericardial tamponade:
  • Malignancy: ~50% of cases
  • Viral/idiopathic pericarditis: ~15% of cases
  • Renal failure/uremia: ~10% of cases
Other causes include:
  • Acute MI (with ventricular rupture)
  • Aortic dissection with rupture into the pericardial space
  • Chest trauma
  • Complication of coronary angioplasty or cardiac surgery

O **Review vital signs**

Hypotension and tachycardia are hallmarks of tamponade.
Check for *pulsus paradoxus* (>10 mm Hg fall in systolic BP with inspiration).
  • Measure pulsus paradox with standard BP cuff, deflating slowly. Korotkoff sounds will initially be heard only during expiration. With further deflation, sounds heard throughout respiratory cycle.
    • Difference between systolic BP at which first Korotkoff sound is heard and when all sounds are heard is the pulsus paradox.
  • May also be increased with severe chronic obstructive pulmonary disease, asthma, acute pulmonary embolism.

Perform a focused physical examination
Jugular venous pressure (JVP): Routinely elevated in tamponade (due to increased right atrial pressure), unless the patient is dehydrated. Rarely, Kussmaul's sign is present (paradoxical increase in JVP during inspiration).
Cardiac: Diminished heart sounds. A pericardial rub may be present.
Beck's triad: elevated JVP, hypotension, quiet heart sounds.
  • Classic physical findings of tamponade.

Review chest radiograph
Cardiomegaly with a globular cardiac silhouette ("water bottle heart").
The lung fields are usually clear, unless there is concomitant lung disease.

Obtain an electrocardiogram
With large effusions, may see electrical alternans (alternating QRS axis) due to the heart's rhythmic motion within the pericardial sac.
Low QRS voltage is common.
Look for evidence of myocardial infarction or pericarditis (ST elevations).

A Pericardial tamponade

Pathophysiology
Normally the pericardial space contains less than 50 cc of lubricating fluid. As fluid accumulates in the pericardial space, the intrapericardial pressure rises and compresses the cardiac chambers, thus impairing cardiac filling. This results in a rise in JVP and a fall in cardiac output.
Tamponade may develop if greater than 200 cc of fluid accumulates rapidly. Slowly progressive effusions may reach 1 to 2 L before tamponade occurs.

Differential diagnosis
- Acute myocardial infarction (especially right ventricular infarction)
- Aortic dissection   - Acute pulmonary embolism
- Tension pneumothorax   - Congestive heart failure

P Admit patient to the ICU

Perform an emergent echocardiogram in any patient suspected of having tamponade
Will confirm the presence of a pericardial effusion.
Can demonstrate compression of cardiac chambers (atrial and/or ventricular collapse) and impairment of ventricular filling.

Support blood pressure in hypotensive patients
Give intravenous fluids and vasopressors (i.e., dopamine, phenylephrine) while awaiting pericardiocentesis.

Perform emergent pericardiocentesis in patients with confirmed tamponade
Performed percutaneously by inserting a needle into the pericardial space from a subxiphoid approach.
Removal of 10 to 20 cc of fluid may be enough to restore hemodynamic stability.
A catheter can be left in the pericardial space for 24 to 48 hours to allow continuous drainage of fluid.
If tamponade is the result of myocardial infarction (ventricular rupture) or aortic dissection, only the minimal amount of fluid needed to restore adequate BP should be drained and an emergent cardiothoracic surgery consult should be called for.
• Removal of a greater volume may increase flow of blood into the pericardium and induce abrupt hemodynamic collapse.
Send fluid for culture and cytology.

Consider right heart catheterization in stable patients in whom the diagnosis is suspected but not confirmed on echocardiogram
Reveals equilibration of right atrial, right ventricular, and pulmonary capillary wedge pressures during diastole.

Consult cardiothoracic surgery if the effusion rapidly reaccumulates after drainage
Consider partial resection of the pericardium ("pericardial window").
• Allows fluid to drain into the left thoracic cavity and prevents recurrent tamponade.

S **What are the patient's symptoms?**

Patients most often present with symptoms of right-sided heart failure:
- Lethargy and fatigue
- Dyspnea
- Abdominal fullness
- Peripheral edema

Right upper-quadrant tenderness (secondary to liver congestion).

Diagnosis is often delayed because initial symptoms are often nonspecific (lethargy and fatigue). Other symptoms occur later in the disease.

Does the patient have factors that would predispose to pericardial constriction?

History of acute pericarditis

Tuberculosis (TB)
- Most common cause of pericardial constriction worldwide

History of carcinoma or of radiation therapy to the chest

Connective tissue diseases (e.g., systemic lupus, rheumatoid arthritis)

Previous cardiac surgery

 Review vital signs

Pulsus paradox is present in ~15% of patients with constriction.

Perform a thorough cardiac examination, looking for

Elevated JVP with prominent X and Y descents.

Kussmaul's sign.
- Failure of the jugular venous pressure (JVP) to fall (or a paradoxical increase in JVP) with inspiration.

Pericardial knock.
- A high-pitched third heart sound, caused by the rapid cessation of ventricular filling in early diastole (see "Pathophysiology" below).

Assess for other signs of right heart failure
- Ascites
- Lower extremity edema
- Pleural effusion
- Hepatomegaly (secondary to liver congestion)

Obtain a chest radiogram

Cardiac size is usually normal (as opposed to enlarged with tamponade).

Calcification of the pericardium may be apparent.

Look for evidence of prior TB.

Obtain an electrocardiogram

Low QRS voltage may be seen and atrial fibrillation is commonly present.

 Constrictive pericarditis

A condition in which the visceral and parietal layers of the pericardium become adherent, thickened, and fibrotic, resulting in impairment of ventricular filling in diastole.

Pathophysiology

The thickened pericardium forms a rigid shell around the heart. Early diastolic filling of the heart occurs normally but abruptly stops when the volume of the heart reaches the constraints of the pericardium. Intracardiac pressure then rises equally in all chambers.

Etiologies
Can occur after pericarditis from any cause, most commonly:
- Infectious (e.g., TB, viral, fungal)
- Trauma: cardiac surgery
- Idiopathic
- Neoplastic (lung, breast)
- Radiation induced
- Connective tissue disorders

Differential diagnosis
- Restrictive cardiomyopathy
- Right ventricle infarction
- Cor-pulmonale
- Cardiac tamponade
- Pulmonary hypertension

P **Obtain noninvasive study to confirm the diagnosis**
Echocardiography is the initial test of choice.
- May visualize the thickened pericardium.
- Reveals a leftward shift of the interventricular septum with inspiration.
- Doppler techniques reveal normal early diastolic LV function and helps differentiate from restrictive cardiomyopathy.

Consider obtaining a cardiac computed tomography (CT) or magnetic resonance imaging (MRI) if echocardiography not confirmatory.
- More sensitive for identifying pericardial thickening (MRI) and calcification (CT). May reveal evidence of constrictive physiology.

Consider cardiac catheterization if diagnosis not established by noninvasive means
This is the gold standard for diagnosis.
Hemodynamic findings include:
- Elevated right atrial pressure.
- Rapid x and y descent in the right atrial pressure tracing.
- Inspiratory increase in right atrial pressure (Kussmaul's sign).
- Rapid early diastolic filling of the ventricles followed by a plateau in the ventricular diastolic pressure ("dip and plateau sign").
- Equilibration of left ventricle and right ventricle diastolic pressure.

Treat congestive symptoms
Use loop diuretics to control edema.
- Furosemide 20 mg daily. Increase up to 200 mg twice daily if needed.
Consider adding spironolactone for patients with ascites.
Place on sodium restricted diet (<2.0 gm/day).

Check PPD to rule out TB

Refer to cardiothoracic surgery if symptoms persist despite medical therapy
Consider surgical removal of the pericardium ("pericardial stripping").
- Is the definitive therapy for constrictive pericarditis.
- Operative mortality may be as high as 10% (higher in patients with radiation-induced pericardial constriction, and in patients with advanced age, renal insufficiency, or ventricular dysfunction).
- 80% to 90% of patients will improve significantly after this procedure.

S **What are the patient's current symptoms?**
Chest pain that is identical to other causes of pericarditis.
- Usually sharp, substernal, and moderate to severe in intensity.
- Pleuritic (worse with deep inspiration).
- Positional (worse when lying down).
- May radiate to the shoulder or scapula.
- May be associated with dyspnea.

Systemic symptoms are more common than with other forms of pericarditis.
- Fevers   • Myalgias   • Malaise

Has the patient recently had a condition that predisposes to Dressler's syndrome?
Myocardial infarction.
Cardiac surgery.
- "Post-pericardiotomy syndrome."
Pulmonary embolism.
- 3% to 4% of patients develop a Dressler's-like syndrome, presumably resulting from pleural infarction and subsequent pleuro-pericarditis.

How long after the myocardial infarction or cardiac surgery did the symptoms develop?
Inflammatory pericarditis is common in the first several days after an MI or cardiac surgery – this does not constitute Dressler's syndrome.
Dressler's syndrome or post-pericardiotomy syndrome occurs weeks to months after the initial event.

O **Review vital signs**
Fever is almost always present (up to 104° F).

The presence of tachycardia, hypotension, and elevated pulsus paradox should raise the suspicion for pericardial tamponade. (See SOAP 20.)

Perform a focused physical examination looking for
Jugular venous distention: reflects elevated right atrial pressure and may indicate accumulation of pericardial fluid.

A pericardial rub is pathognomonic for pericarditis.
- A coarse, scratching sound heard best with the diaphragm of the stethoscope and with the patient leaning forward.
- Classically has three components reflecting atrial systole, ventricular systole, and ventricular diastole.

A pleural rub or evidence of a pleural effusion may be present.

Obtain an electrocardiogram
The classic changes of pericarditis are often not present.

Low QRS voltage and electrical alternans may be seen if there is a large pericardial effusion.

Review laboratory data
White blood cell count is frequently elevated.
An elevated erythrocyte sedimentation rate is almost always present (often >100).
C-reactive protein and other markers of inflammation are elevated.

Dressler's syndrome

Dressler's syndrome is an autoimmune-mediated, inflammatory pericarditis that occurs weeks to months after a myocardial infarction. A similar process can occur after cardiac surgery (termed "post-pericardiotomy syndrome").

Pathogenesis

Cardiac injury releases myocardial antigens that stimulate antibodies to form. These are deposited in the pericardium and pleura and elicit an inflammatory response. The degree of tissue infarction correlates with the occurrence of Dressler's syndrome.

Differential diagnosis

- Post-infarction pericarditis (occurs days after an MI)
  - Infectious pericarditis
  - Angina
  - Pleurisy
  - Costochondritis
  - Pulmonary embolism
  - Myocardial infarction
  - Pneumonia
  - Post-sternotomy pain or infection

Prognosis

Usually self-limited, but occasionally associated with pericardial tamponade or constriction.
Occasionally can become recurrent.

P **Obtain a chest radiograph**

Pleural effusions are often present.
An enlarged cardiac silhouette will be seen if there is a significant pericardial effusion.

Consider obtaining an echocardiogram

Assess the presence and size of a pericardial effusion.
Exclude pericardial tamponade.

Start anti-inflammatory agents

NSAIDs are the treatment of choice.
  - Ibuprofen 400 to 800 mg tid OR.
  - Indomethacin 25 to 50 mg tid OR.
  - Aspirin 2–6 gm/day.
Colchicine 0.6 mg bid may be added, especially for recurrent pericarditis.
If symptoms are refractory to NSAIDs, steroids are usually effective.
  - Prednisone 60 mg daily tapered over 1 to 2 weeks.
  - Should be used with caution as they can delay myocardial healing after myocardial infarction or wound healing after cardiac surgery.

S **Does the patient have symptoms attributable to mitral stenosis (MS)?**
Common presenting symptoms include:
- Dyspnea   • Palpitations   • Chest pain   • Fatigue   • Hemoptysis
- Hoarseness (Ortner syndrome): recurrent laryngeal nerve compression by the pulmonary artery

Symptoms of MS are often exertional and usually start in the third or fourth decade of life.
Patients with MS may also present with the following complications:
- Atrial fibrillation
- Systemic embolic events including stroke and ischemic digits
- Symptoms of left or right heart failure (orthopnea, paroxysmal nocturnal dyspnea, edema, etc)
- Infective endocarditis (see SOAP 28)

Obtain a medical history
Rheumatic fever is the most common cause of mitral stenosis.

Obtain a thorough review of systems

O **Check vital signs**
An irregularly irregular pulse indicates atrial fibrillation.
Tachycardia is poorly tolerated in patients with significant MS.

Perform a cardiovascular examination looking for signs of MS
Mitral facies (a plethoric, blush-like appearance over the face).
Left parasternal (right ventricular) heave—indicates pulmonary hypertension.
Loud first heart sound (S_1).
- The mitral valve closes from a maximally open position.

Loud P_2 (pulmonic component of the second heart sound).
- Indicates pulmonary hypertension.

An opening snap of the valve may be appreciated following the second heart sound.
Murmur: low-pitched, mid-diastolic rumble.
- Best heard with the bell of a stethoscope over the point of maximal intensity with the patient in a left lateral position and in expiration.
- Presystolic accentuation of the murmur occurs when sinus rhythm is present.

Graham Steele murmur: pulmonary regurgitation murmur due to pulmonary HTN.
Listen for associated aortic and tricuspid valve disease.

Perform a pulmonary examination
Presence of crackles may indicate pulmonary edema.

Obtain an electrocardiogram
Left atrial enlargement (P mitrale; P wave >1 mm deep in V_1, >120 msec long in II).
Right ventricular hypertrophy (indicates associated pulmonary HTN).
Often in atrial fibrillation.

Obtain a chest radiograph
Left atrial and pulmonary artery enlargement without cardiac dilation is suggestive of MS.
Check for evidence of pulmonary edema or pulmonary HTN.

A **Mitral stenosis**

Pathophysiology
Scarring of the mitral valve results in progressive narrowing of the valve orifice and development of a transvalvular pressure gradient, resulting in increased left atrial

and pulmonary venous pressures. Tachycardia shortens diastole, further impairing transmitral flow and increasing left atrial and pulmonary pressures.

Etiology
Rheumatic fever (99% of cases): due to antigenic mimicry between a group A beta hemolytic streptococcus and the mitral valve, resulting in fibrosis and scarring of the valve with leaflet fusion, shortening of the chordae, and narrowing of the valvular orifice.
Degenerative calcification of the valve and annulus.

Severity classified by valve area
- Normal: 4 to 6 cm^2
- Moderate stenosis: 1.0 to 1.5 cm^2
- Mild stenosis: 1.5 to 2.5 cm^2
- Severe stenosis: <1.0 cm^2

Differential diagnosis
Atrial myxoma

P

Obtain an echocardiogram
Confirm the diagnosis of MS and assess its severity; assess other valves.
Evaluate for potential balloon valvuloplasty.

Consider cardiac catheterization
Confirm the severity of the MS if not clarified by echocardiography.
Measure pulmonary pressure.
Assess for concomitant coronary artery disease: may require coronary artery bypass graft at valve surgery.
- Angiography is performed in all patients with risk factors or older than 40 years of age.

Institute medical therapy for MS
Control HR with AV nodal agents (digoxin, beta-blockers, calcium channel blockers).
Diuretics to control congestive symptoms.
Restore and maintain normal sinus rhythm when possible.
Anticoagulation for atrial fibrillation (goal INR: 2.5–3.5).
Antibiotic prophylaxis for infective endocarditis and recurrent rheumatic fever.

Consider surgical options in appropriate patients
Candidates for surgical approaches to treatment include:
- Mitral valve area less than 1 cm^2 (regardless of symptoms).
- Symptoms despite medical therapy in patients with MV area 1 to 1.5 cm^2.
- Patients with MS and embolic events.
- Before pregnancy with severe MS; during pregnancy if CHF develops.
- Asymptomatic patients with moderate to severe MS and recent onset AF.
Surgical options include:
- Mitral balloon valvuloplasty (least invasive technique).
  - Procedure of choice in eligible patients with pliable, minimally thickened, or calcified valves, without significant chordal thickening.
- Mitral valve repair: excellent outcome in those who are suitable (95% survival at 10 yrs and 90% freedom from operation).
- Mitral valve replacement.
  - Tissue valves or mechanical valves are available.
  - Choice of valve depends on (1) patient's age (tissue valves last ~10 years), (2) bleeding risk (mechanical valves require life-long anticoagulation), (3) patient choice.

S Does the patient have symptoms attributable to aortic stenosis (AS)?

The classic presenting symptoms of AS include:
- Angina
- Dyspnea
- Syncope

Other symptoms include:
- Palpitations (arrhythmias)
- Orthopnea (heart failure)
- Paroxysmal nocturnal dyspnea
- Dizziness, presyncope

Symptoms of AS are often exertional.

Obtain a medical history
Aortic coarctation: frequently associated with a bicuspid aortic valve.
Rheumatic fever.
Childhood murmur: may suggest congenital AS.

Obtain a thorough review of symptoms

O **Check vital signs**
A narrow pulse pressure may be present in severe aortic stenosis.

Perform a cardiovascular examination, looking for signs of aortic stenosis
Point of maximal impulse.
- Sustained (left ventricular [LV] heave) due to LV pressure overload.
- Displaced when LV failure is present.

Systolic ejection murmur.
- Heard best at the right sternal border, second intercostal space.
- Peaks later in systole with more severe AS.
- Accentuated by squatting (increases venous return), and reduced by standing or during sustained Valsalva (decreases venous return).
- Radiates to the carotid arteries.
- May radiate to the LV apex and mimic MR (Gallavardin phenomenon).

Low volume, slow rising carotid pulses (pulsus parvus et tardus) indicate severe AS.
Second heart sound goes from normally split (A_2 preceding P_2) in mild stenosis to paradoxically split (A_2 following P_2) in severe stenosis. A_2 is often soft and may disappear as the valve narrows.
An S_4 is often present.

Perform a pulmonary examination
Crackles may indicate presence of pulmonary edema/congestive heart failure.

Obtain an ECG looking for evidence of significant aortic stenosis
Left ventricular hypertrophy with strain pattern (present in 85% of AS).
Left atrial enlargement (present in 80% of AS).
Various degrees of heart block (present in 5% of AS) may result from severe calcification around the AV, or, if the valve is infected, annular abscess formation.

Obtain a chest radiograph
Calcification of the aortic valve.
Post-stenotic dilation of the ascending aorta may be present.

 Aortic stenosis

Pathophysiology
Normal AV area: 3 to 4 cm^2. Disease of the AV produces progressive valvular obstruction resulting in LV hypertrophy, decreased cardiac output, and progressive LV failure.

Severity classified by valve area
Mild: AV area 1.0 to 2.0 cm^2
Moderate: AV area 0.8 to 1.0 cm^2
Severe: AV area <0.8 cm^2 or mean pressure gradient >45 mm Hg

Prognosis/survival of untreated patients after onset of symptoms
    - CHF: 1 to 2 years   - Syncope: 3 years   - Angina: 5 years

Etiology
Bicuspid aortic valve: presents with AS at age 20 to 40 years
Rheumatic heart disease: presents with AS at age 40 to 50 years
Senile calcific disease: presents with AS at age 50 to 70 years

Differential diagnosis
Hypertrophic cardiomyopathy with an LV outflow tract gradient
Subvalvular or supravalvular aortic stenosis
Mitral regurgitation (AS murmur may mimic MR)

P **Obtain an echocardiogram to confirm the diagnosis**
Can visualize the restriction of motion of the valve leaflets and determine the mechanism of AS (bicuspid valve, rheumatic disease, etc.).
Doppler techniques can quantify the severity of AS.
Exclude other associated valvular disease.
Assess left ventricular function.

Consider cardiac catheterization
Confirm AS severity if clinical questions persist after echocardiography.
Assess coronary anatomy: may require concomitant coronary artery bypass surgery at the time of valve replacement surgery.

Obtain serial echocardiograms and clinical evaluations in asymptomatic patients
Patients with mild AS should have a repeat echocardiogram every 1 to 2 years.
Patients with moderate or severe asymptomatic AS should have echocardiograms and clinical assessment of symptoms every 6 months.

Consider starting lipid-lowering therapy (with statins)
May delay progression of degenerative AS.

Refer all symptomatic patients for valve replacement surgery
There is no effective medical treatment for severe or symptomatic AS.
Replacement of the AV should be considered in patients with:
- Symptomatic AS (even if valve area is not in the severe range).
- Severe AS (valve area <0.8 cm^2), even without symptoms.
- Rapidly progressive stenosis on serial echocardiographs (even without symptoms).
- Valvular complications including bacterial endocarditis.

Tissue valves (cadaveric, bovine, or porcine) or mechanical valves are available.
Choice of prosthetic valve type depends on:
- Patient's age (tissue valves last ~10 years).
- Bleeding risk (mechanical valves require chronic anticoagulation).
- Patient choice.

Prescribe antibiotic prophylaxis to prevent endocarditis in all patients with AS

S **Does the patient have symptoms attributable to mitral regurgitation (MR)?**
Common presenting symptoms include:

- Dyspnea
- Decreased exercise tolerance
- Paroxysmal nocturnal dyspnea
- Fatigue
- Orthopnea

Occasionally patients present with symptoms related to infective endocarditis or myocardial infarction, both of which can cause acute MR.

Does the patient have a condition that predisposes to MR?
- Mitral valve leaflet prolapse
- Dilated cardiomyopathy
- Myocardial infarction (MI)
- Infective endocarditis (IE)
- Connective tissue disorders

Obtain a medical history: does the patient have a history of:
- Rheumatic fever
- Use of anorexigenic drugs (i.e., phentermine-fenfluramine)
- Recent dental work

O **Check vital signs**
Patients with acute MR are frequently tachycardic, hypotensive, and in respiratory distress.

Perform a cardiovascular examination looking for signs of MR
On palpation:
- The point of maximal intensity (PMI) is hyperdynamic in acute MR, and diffuse when the LV is dilated.
- Left parasternal (right ventricular) heave indicates pulmonary hypertension.

On auscultation:
- Soft first heart sound (S_1).
  - This is in contrast to mitral stenosis where S_1 is loud.
- Loud P_2 (pulmonic component of the second heart sound).
  - Indicates pulmonary hypertension.
- Murmur:
  - Holosystolic murmur best heard during expiration, at the area of the PMI, using the diaphragm of the stethoscope, with the patient in the left lateral position.
  - Classically radiates to the axilla, rarely to the left parasternal area.
  - With mitral valve prolapse, there is a mid systolic click and a late systolic murmur.
- An S_3 is frequently present in severe MR.
- Listen carefully for associated mitral stenosis or aortic valve disease.

Listen for evidence of pulmonary edema

Obtain an electrocardiogram
Look for evidence of ischemia, especially in acute MR.
For known chronic MR look for the presence of left atrial enlargement.
- P mitrale; P wave >1 mm deep in V_1 and >120 msec long in lead II.
Atrial fibrillation is common.

Obtain a chest radiograph
Left atrial or left ventricular dilation is usually present, and pulmonary vascular congestion is common.

A **Mitral regurgitation**

Pathophysiology

In acute MR, LV function is usually normal. The sudden regurgitation of blood into the left atrium results in an acute increase in left atrial (LA) pressure, which is transmitted to the pulmonary vasculature resulting in pulmonary edema. In chronic MR, the LA and left ventricle (LV) gradually dilate to accommodate the excess volume; congestive heart failure (CHF) occurs after LV dysfunction develops.

Classifying the mechanism of MR

Primary valvular MR: relates to a diseased valve (MVP, rheumatic disease, endocarditis, papillary muscle infarction occurring with an MI).

Functional MR: regurgitation occurring in the presence of normal valve leaflets (e.g., from dilation of the mitral valve annulus due to cardiomyopathy).

Differential diagnosis of MR murmur

- Tricuspid regurgitation
- Hypertrophic obstructive cardiomyopathy
- Ventricular septal defect

P **Obtain an echocardiogram**

Confirm the diagnosis and assess the severity of MR.
- Graded 0 (no MR) to 4+ (severe MR).

Assess LV and RV size function.

Assess mechanism of MR and evaluate for other associated valve disease.

Obtain cardiology evaluation for all patients with more than mild MR

Require serial echocardiograms and examinations to assess MR progression.
- Evaluate symptom status, MR severity, LV size, and LV function.

Empiric treatment with angiotensin-converting enzyme inhibitors (ACEI) or diuretics is not indicated —*may mask the development of LV dysfunction and delay consideration of surgical therapies.*

Consider right and left heart catheterization in patients with severe MR

Measure pulmonary pressures and confirm severity of MR.
- Tall V waves in the pulmonary pressure tracing indicate severe MR.

Assess for concomitant coronary artery disease that may require surgical revascularization (coronary artery bypass grafting) at valve surgery.

Refer all patients with symptomatic MR for valve surgery

Surgical options include:
- Annuloplasty ring: restores normal mitral annular size.
- Mitral valve repair: used most commonly for mitral valve prolapse.
- Mitral valve replacement: used in patients with non-repairable valves.
- Mechanical valves or bioprosthetic valves are available.

Patients with severe LV dysfunction, right heart failure, or severe concomitant medical issues may be poor candidates for surgery.

Medical management of patients with symptomatic MR who are not surgical candidates is similar to that for other causes of CHF (diuretics, ACEI, digoxin).

Consider valve surgery in all patients with moderate/severe MR on echocardiogram and any of the following features

- Any degree of CHF
- LV dilatation (LV internal dimensions in systole >45 mm)
- Left ventricular ejection fraction <60%

Prescribe antibiotic prophylaxis to prevent endocarditis in patients with more than mild MR

S **Does the patient have symptoms attributable to aortic insufficiency (AI)?**
Common symptoms of *chronic AI* include:
- Prominent heart beat/palpitations   • Atypical chest pain
- Symptoms of congestive heart failure (dyspnea on exertion, orthopnea, paroxysmal nocturnal dyspnea, and lower extremity edema)

Common symptoms of *acute AI* include:
- Acute dyspnea   • Syncope   • Cardiovascular collapse

Does the patient have any condition that predisposes to AI?
- Known aortic aneurysm   - Prior or acute aortic dissection   - Endocarditis
- Prior rheumatic fever   - Ankylosing spondylitis   - Prior syphilis
- Collagen vascular disorders (e.g., Marfan's, Ehlers-Danlos syndrome)
- Congenital bicuspid aortic valve

O **Check vital signs**
Chronic AI is associated with hypertension and a widened pulse pressure.
Patients with acute AI are usually tachycardic, tachypneic, and hypotensive.

Perform a cardiovascular examination looking for signs of AI
On inspection:
- Quincke's sign: cyclic blushing and blanching of capillary nail beds.
- Corrigan's pulse or Water hammer pulse: prominent carotid systolic pulsation that collapses during diastole.
- De Musset's sign: head bobbing with each heartbeat.
- Muller's sign: pulsation of the uvula with each heartbeat.

On palpation:
- The point of maximal impulse is diffuse, hyperdynamic, and may be displaced inferolaterally.

On cardiac auscultation:
- AI causes a diastolic decrescendo murmur heard best along the left sternal border, with the patient sitting forward, and at end inspiration.

  • In acute AI, the murmur may not be appreciated whereas in chronic AI the murmur may last through all of diastole.

- An aortic systolic murmur is usually present (due to increased stroke volume).
- Austin-Flint murmur: a mid diastolic murmur at the PMI that mimics mitral stenosis. Represents fluttering of the mitral valve leaflet within the AI jet.
- S_1 is often soft due to premature mitral valve closure and A_2 is soft or absent.

On vascular examination:
- Duroziez's sign: systolic and diastolic femoral bruits heard when the artery is partially compressed.
- Traube's sign: "pistol shot" sound heard on auscultation of the femoral artery.

Look for signs of congestive heart failure

Look for signs of the predisposing conditions listed above

Obtain an electrocardiogram
Often normal aside from sinus tachycardia.
In acute AI from aortic dissection, ischemic ECG changes may be present.

A

Aortic insufficiency

Pathophysiology

AI is a volume overload state. The increased LV volume causes an increased stroke volume resulting in systolic hypertension. The backflow of blood into the LV during diastole results in a low diastolic blood pressure. The resulting widened pulse pressure causes most of the findings on physical examination. Chronic volume overload leads to LV dilation and eventually LV failure.

Etiology

Valvular abnormalities:

- Connective tissue disorders (i.e., ankylosing spondylitis).
- Inflammatory: rheumatic fever.
- Infective: endocarditis.
- Mechanical: bicuspid aortic valve, aortic dissection.

Aortic abnormalities (causes AI by distorting the aortic valve):

- Cystic medial necrosis: Marfan's syndrome.
- Inflammatory: aortitis secondary to syphilis.
- Mechanical: severe hypertension, ascending aortic aneurysm.

P

Obtain an echocardiogram

Assess the mechanism and severity of AI and assess LV size and function.
Assess for disease of other valves.

Obtain a chest radiograph

Evaluate for LV dilation, aortic aneurysm, and evidence of pulmonary edema.

Refer patients with greater than mild AI to cardiology to assist with management

Asymptomatic patients with mild to moderate AI require no specific therapy.
Asymptomatic patients with moderate to severe AI and normal LV function should receive afterload reduction with nifedipine or angiotensin-converting enzyme inhibitors.

- May delay onset of symptoms and reduce the need for surgery.

Avoid β-blockers, calcium channel blockers, and digoxin.

- Bradycardia worsens AI by allowing more time for regurgitation.

Medical management is only appropriate for patients with AI who are asymptomatic and have normal LV size and function.

Perform serial examinations and echocardiography to determine the timing of valve surgery

Perform every 1 to 2 years in patients with mild to moderate AI.
Perform every 6 months in patients with severe, although asymptomatic, AI.

Consider cardiac catheterization

Can clarify the severity of AI if questions persist after echocardiography.
Assess for concomitant coronary artery disease before valve replacement surgery.

Consider aortic valve replacement

In any patient with moderate or severe AI who has CHF.
In acute severe AI from any cause (e.g., dissection, endocarditis).
In asymptomatic patients with moderate to severe AI with echo revealing:

- Evidence of a dilating LV (LV end systolic dimension >55 mm) *OR*
- Abnormal LV systolic function (LVEF <55%).

Prescribe antibiotic prophylaxis to prevent endocarditis in all patients with AI

S **Does the patient have symptoms attributable to tricuspid regurgitation (TR)?**
Many patients with TR have no specific symptoms. When present, symptoms are
often attributable to right-sided heart failure:
- Fatigue and lethargy
- Neck fullness
- Increasing abdominal girth with ascites
- Dyspnea
- Lower extremity edema

Obtain a medical history
- Rheumatic fever/rheumatic heart disease
- Congenital heart disease (e.g., Epstein's anomaly, pulmonary stenosis)
- Blunt chest trauma
- Prior endocarditis
- Prior inferior myocardial infarction

Does the patient have other risk factors for developing TR?
IV drug use can lead to tricuspid valve endocarditis.
Any condition that causes pulmonary hypertension can result in right ventricular
dilation and secondary TR.
- Left-sided heart failure.
- Primary pulmonary hypertension.
- Pulmonary emboli.
- Chronic obstructive pulmonary disease.

Perform a cardiovascular examination
O Classically the jugular venous pressure is significantly elevated with a single promi-
nent waveform ("CV" wave).
A left parasternal heave (right ventricular heave) is usually present.
The murmur of TR is holosystolic, best heard over the fifth intercostal space at the
left or right sternal edge, and increases in intensity with inspiration.
- May be confused with mitral regurgitation (MR), but MR is heard best over the
left ventricular (LV) apex (point of maximal impulse) and radiates to the axilla,
whereas TR does not.
A loud P_2 component of the second heart sound confirms the presence of
pulmonary hypertension.

Look for evidence of left- and right-sided heart failure
Pulmonary crackles or pulmonary effusions.
An enlarged, pulsatile liver is commonly present with severe TR.
Ascites.
Lower extremity edema.

Review the electrocardiogram
Right atrial enlargement (P wave >1 mm high in V_1; >2.5 mm high in lead II).
Right ventricular enlargement (RsR' in lead V_1 with right axis deviation).

Obtain a chest radiograph
Review for cardiomegaly, pleural effusions, evidence of lung disease.

A **Tricuspid regurgitation**
Regurgitation of blood across the TV during systole. When severe, causes elevation of right atrial and systemic venous pressures resulting in right heart failure.

Causes of TR
Primary valvular abnormality/dysfunction:
- Rheumatic heart disease (20% to 30% of cases).
- Endocarditis.
- Tricuspid valve prolapse (usually seen with mitral valve prolapse).
- Blunt chest trauma with papillary muscle rupture.
- Carcinoid syndrome with involvement of the TV.
- Ebstein's anomaly: displacement of the tricuspid valve annulus into the right ventricle causing malcoaptation of the tricuspid leaflets.

Secondary TR resulting from right ventricular dilation/dysfunction:
- Pulmonary hypertension (primary or secondary).
- RV infarction.
- Congenital heart disease (e.g., pulmonic stenosis, Tetralogy of Fallot).

P **Obtain an echocardiogram**
Confirm the diagnosis of TR and assess its severity.
Assess RV size and function.
Assess mechanism of TR (? primary valve abnormality or secondary TR).
Estimate pulmonary artery pressure to evaluate for pulmonary hypertension.
- Estimated from the velocity of the TR jet (pressure = $4 \times \text{velocity}^2$).
- May be inaccurate with severe TR (underestimates true PA pressure).

Obtain blood cultures if endocarditis is suspected

Use loop diuretics to control/reduce congestive symptoms
Furosemide 20 to 200 mg once or twice daily may be needed.
Nitrates may further improve symptoms by reducing preload and lowering pulmonary arterial pressures; use with caution in patients with RV failure.

Evaluate for pulmonary disease in patients with pulmonary hypertension
Obtain pulmonary function tests and arterial blood gas (on room air).
Consider ventilation-perfusion scan or computed tomography scan to exclude pulmonary embolic disease.

Consider right heart catheterization
Measure right heart and pulmonary pressures and confirm the severity of TR in patients in whom echocardiography is inadequate.
Tailor management of vasodilator therapy in patients with pulmonary hypertension.

Consider vasodilator therapy in patients with primary pulmonary hypertension
    - Epoprostenol   - Sildenafil   - Bosentan

Antibiotic prophylaxis for infective endocarditis

Refer patients to surgery who have
Severe TR resulting from a primary valvular abnormality whose symptoms are uncontrolled on medical therapy.
- Surgery must be performed prior to the development of RV failure.
Surgical options include an annuloplasty ring to return the annulus to a more physiologic size and tricuspid valve replacement.

S **What are the patient's presenting symptoms?**

Signs/symptoms of acute endocarditis include:

- Congestive heart failure
- Sweats/rigors
- Myalgias
- Hemodynamic instability
- Fevers

Symptoms of a more subacute illness include:

- Night sweats
- Malaise
- Abdominal pain
- Arthralgia
- Weight loss

Complications with which patients may present include:

- Embolic: transient ischemic attack/stroke, renal failure, acute myocardial infarction, pulmonary or systemic abscess.
- Vasculitic: hematuria/renal failure, visual obscuration (retinal vasculitis).

Does the patient have risk factors for endocarditis?

Prosthetic heart valves.

Valvular or structural heart disease.

- Bicuspid aortic valve
- Mitral valve prolapse
- Rheumatic heart disease
- Ventricular septal defects. (Atrial septal defects are not a risk factor for endocarditis as blood flow across an atrial shunt is not turbulent.)

Poor dentition or recent dental work.

IV drug use – predisposes to right-sided endocarditis.

Perform a thorough review of systems

May elicit an alternative source of fever.

Recent antibiotic use may affect sensitivities of blood cultures.

O **Examine the patient carefully for manifestations of endocarditis**

Finger clubbing: more often noted in subacute presentations.

Splinter hemorrhages: in the proximal two thirds of the nail bed.

Conjunctival petechiae.

Osler's nodes: white, painful, nodular, lesions on the digits (e.g., finger pulp).

Janeway lesions: painless, red, microhemorrhages on the palms or soles.

Roth spots: Retinal hemorrhages with central clearing.

A new or changing murmur on cardiac examination.

Splenomegaly on abdominal palpation.

Review laboratory tests

Leukocytosis is common.

Hemolytic anemia or anemia of chronic disease is frequently present.

Erythrocyte sedimentation rate is usually elevated (often >100 mm/hr).

A sudden deterioration in renal function may reflect renal emboli.

Hematuria may reflect immune complex glomerulonephritis or renal emboli.

Varying degrees of heart block may be seen on electrocardiogram and often reflects a valve ring abscess with extension of the infection into the conduction system.

Obtain a chest radiograph

Look specifically for pulmonary abscesses, pneumonia or infarction.

Infectious endocarditis
An infection of the cardiac valves. Diagnosis is based on history, physical examination, and laboratory investigations as detailed above. Criteria to assist with the diagnosis (e.g., Von Ryan criteria, Duke criteria, etc) may increase specificity.
Common causative organisms include *Streptococcus viridans* (mouth flora), *Staphylococcus aureus*, and *Enterococcus*.
Fastidious organisms may require long periods of incubation (7–21 days).
- HACEK organisms (*Haemophilus, Actinobacillus, Cardiobacterium, Corynebacterium*, and *Eikenella*).
- *Bartonella, Brucella, Mycoplasma, Legionella, Coxiella* (Q fever).

Differential diagnosis
Noninfectious endocarditis
- Libman-Sachs endocarditis in SLE
- Malignancy
Vasculitic disease
Cardiac myxoma

 Admit to telemetry floor or to the cardiac care unit
Monitor for progressive heart block and hemodynamic instability.

Start empiric antibiotics
Third-generation cephalosporin is the usual empiric therapy.
Use vancomycin if infection with MRSA is suspected.
Consider addition of gentamycin or rifampicin for synergistic effects.

Obtain blood cultures
At least three sets of blood cultures from different sites over several hours are essential. Of note, causative organisms are mostly aerobic in nature.

Obtain an echocardiogram
Modified criteria for diagnosis of endocarditis (e.g., Duke's criteria) now incorporate echo findings in the diagnosis.
Important findings to note on echocardiogram include:
- Presence and size of vegetations (lesions > 1 cm frequently embolize).
- Severity of valvular regurgitation.
Request transthoracic echocardiogram (TTE) initially.
A transesophageal echo should be requested if TTE is nondiagnostic and clinical suspicion is high.

Consider referral for valve replacement in patients who
Fail antibiotic treatment (persistent fevers and positive blood cultures).
Develop a paravalvular abscess.
Have emboli to the brain, kidneys or other major organs.
Develop progressive heart block.
Develop congestive heart failure or hemodynamic compromise.
Have endocarditis of a prosthetic heart valve.
Have infection with *S. aureus* or fungi (e.g., *Candida* sp.).
Have large vegetations (>1 cm).

S **Does the patient have symptoms attributable to the VSD?**
Small congenital ventricular septal defects (VSDs) are frequently asymptomatic, especially in childhood.
Large congenital VSDs may cause left heart failure (i.e., dyspnea) at any age.
Adults often present with palpitations (arrhythmias) or symptoms of chronic right-sided heart failure, including dyspnea, fatigue, and lower extremity edema.
Occasionally patients may present with symptoms of endocarditis (see SOAP 28) or paradoxical emboli.
Acquired VSDs usually present with acute left heart failure and hemodynamic collapse several days after a myocardial infarction.

How was the diagnosis made?
Usually suspected on the basis of physical findings.
Infrequently an incidental finding on echocardiogram.

Does the patient have a condition that is associated with having a VSD?
Congenital VSD: Down's syndrome, Turner's syndrome, Trisomy 13, Trisomy 18, Cri du chat, fetal alcohol syndrome, bicuspid aortic valve, aortic coarctation.
Acquired VSD: Recent or prior myocardial infarction.

Obtain a medical and family history
Adults with congenital VSDs often have a lifelong history of having a murmur.
VSD found in ~3% of first degree relatives of patients with VSDs.

O **Check vital signs including the oxygen saturation**
The BP is usually normal unless ventricular failure occurs.
Low oxygen saturations may indicate the presence of pulmonary hypertension and right-to-left shunting of deoxygenated blood (Eisenmenger's syndrome).

Perform a cardiac examination looking for the following clinical findings
Left parasternal heave secondary to a pressure overloaded right ventricle.
Systolic murmur – varies depending on the size of the VSD.
- Small VSDs maintain a high pressure gradient between the left ventricle (LV) and right ventricle (RV) and produce a loud holosystolic murmur at the left sternal edge (second to fourth intercostal space).
  - May radiate to the right chest or the neck depending on site of VSD.
- Large VSDs result in equalization of pressure in the LV and RV and the murmur becomes crescendo-decrescendo and occurs in early systole only.
The murmur is often accompanied by a prominent precordial thrill.
Pulmonary second sound may be loud due to pulmonary hypertension.
A mitral mid-diastolic murmur may be heard with large shunts due to increased flow.

Obtain an electrocardiogram
Changes of left ventricular hypertrophy (see SOAP 62) and in more advanced cases right ventricular hypertrophy (right axis deviation, RsR' in lead V_1) may be present.
Evidence of a recent myocardial infarction (Q waves, ST-T abnormalities) suggests an acquired VSD.

Obtain a chest radiograph
Classic findings include increased pulmonary markings ("shunt vascularity"), dilated pulmonary arteries, and enlarged left atrium and ventricle.
Pulmonary edema may occur with acute VSD from a myocardial infarction.

A **Ventricular septal defect**
A hole in the interventricular septum that allows blood to flow between the right and left ventricles. Initially, blood is shunted from LV to RV resulting in increased pulmonary blood flow and volume overload of the left heart. When pulmonary hypertension develops, shunting may reverse (right-to-left; "Eisenmenger's syndrome") resulting in hypoxemia.
May be congenital (>90%) or acquired (after an acute myocardial infarction).
Four basic types of congenital VSDs, classified by their location in the septum:
- Membranous defects: Most common. 80% of all VSDs.
- Muscular defects: 5% to 20% of VSDs. May be multiple resulting in the pseudonym "Swiss cheese" septum.
- Inlet defects: Uncommon. Often associated with atrial septal defect or atrioventricular canal defects.
- Supracristal or sub-pulmonary defects: Account for 5% to 7% of cases.

Differential diagnosis
Valvular defects causing systolic murmurs (e.g., mitral regurgitation, aortic stenosis).
Other shunts: patent ductus arteriosus, atrial septal defects. (See SOAP 30.)

P **Obtain an echocardiogram**
Flow across the VSD can be confirmed with color Doppler techniques or after injection of agitated saline ("bubble study").
Can assess the RV size and function, estimate PA pressure, and quantify the shunt (estimate Qp:Qs – pulmonary blood flow [Qp] versus systemic blood flow [Qs]).
Can identify LV infarction in patients suspected of having an acquired VSD.
Can identify other associated congenital abnormalities.

Consider cardiac catheterization
Can confirm the diagnosis by identifying a rise in oxygen saturation in the RV, or by demonstrating flow across the septum after injecting contrast into the LV.
Can identify concomitant coronary artery disease in patients requiring surgical repair of the VSD.

Follow small shunts with serial examinations and echocardiographic assessments
Small VSDs identified in childhood often close spontaneously in the first few years of life and require only conservative medical follow up in this period.
- 25% to 50% close spontaneously (60% of these by 3 years of age, 80% by 8 years).
Small VSDs identified in adulthood usually require no specific therapy.
- Features predictive of a benign course include lack of symptoms, normal pulmonary artery pressure, Qp:Qs <1.5:1, no associated valvular disease, normal ventricular size and function.

Consider surgical closure of large VSDs
Large VSDs identified in childhood usually require surgical repair, especially if associated with other cardiac abnormalities.
Large defects identified in adulthood rarely close spontaneously, especially if the Qp:Qs is >2:1.

Refer all VSDs occurring after an MI for emergent surgical repair
These VSDs are associated with a very high morbidity rate even with repair.
Prescribe antibiotic prophylaxis to prevent endocarditis for all patients with VSDs.

Does the patient have any symptoms?

Many patients who have an atrial septal defect (ASD) are asymptomatic.
Common presenting symptoms include:

- Dyspnea
- Palpitations
- Symptoms of right-sided heart failure (e.g., fatigue, pedal edema)

Rarely patients may present with stroke from a paradoxical embolism.

How was the diagnosis originally made?

Often suspected on the basis of physical examination, electrocardiogramy, or chest radiograph.

Frequently noted incidentally on an echocardiogram performed for a different reason.

Does the patient have any other congenital disorders?

Increased incidence of ASD in patients with other congenital heart disease and with Down's syndrome.

O   Obtain the patient's vital signs, including oxygen saturation

Low oxygen saturation in the face of an ASD suggests right-to-left interatrial shunting of deoxygenated blood.

Frequent ectopy and atrial tachyarrhythmias are common in patients with large ASDs.

Perform a physical examination, looking for the following features

Cardiac

- Left parasternal heave (right ventricular [RV] enlargement).
- Systolic ejection murmur (increased flow across the pulmonary valve).
- Characteristically the second heart sound is widely split and does not vary with respiration (fixed split).
- A mid diastolic rumble over the tricuspid area suggests a large shunt.
- A loud P_2 suggests pulmonary hypertension.

Abdomen

- Ascites and hepatomegaly are suggestive of right-sided heart failure.

Extremities

- Bilateral lower extremity edema also suggests right-sided failure.
- Digital clubbing and cyanosis suggest Eisenmenger's syndrome (pulmonary hypertension resulting in right-to-left shunting).

Obtain an electrocardiogram

An incomplete right bundle branch block and left anterior fascicular block are often present with ostium premium defects.

An RsR' pattern in lead V_1 is often present with ostium secundum defects.

Right atrial enlargement (P pulmonale) and right ventricular hypertrophy may be seen if pulmonary hypertension is present.

Atrial arrhythmias including atrial fibrillation and atrial flutter are often present.

Obtain a chest radiograph

May reveal evidence of pulmonary hypertension, increased pulmonary vascularity, right and/or left atrial enlargement, and right ventricular enlargement.

A   Atrial septal defect

Malformation of the interatrial septum results in an abnormal communication between the left and right atria. Interatrial shunting of blood occurs, the direction of which is determined by the pressure difference between the atria. Initial left-to-right shunting results in RV volume overload and dilation, progressive pulmonary hypertension, and eventually right ventricular failure. When right atrial pressure rises above left atrial pressure, right-to-left shunting with resultant hypoxemia occurs (Eisenmenger's syndrome).

Shunts are considered significant when pulmonary flow (Qp) exceeds systemic flow (Qs) by >50% (i.e., Qp:Qs > 1.5:1).

ASDs are classified by their location:
- Ostium premium (20% of cases): involve the endocardial cushion.
  - Associated with a cleft mitral valve leaflet.
- Ostium secundum (70% of cases): occur in the region of the foramen ovale.
- Sinus venosus (10% of cases): occur in the superior aspect of the septum.
  - Associated with anomalous pulmonary venous return.

Differential diagnosis
Patent foramen ovale: normally formed atrial septum but without foraminal closure.
Right-sided valvular defects causing systolic murmurs (e.g., tricuspid regurgitation or pulmonic stenosis).
Other intracardiac shunts: ventricular septal defects (see SOAP 29) and patent ductus arteriosus.

P

Obtain an echocardiogram
Can confirm the diagnosis (with color Doppler or bubble study), assess RV size and function, estimate pulmonary artery (PA) pressure, and quantify shunt (estimate Qp:Qs).
Transesophageal echo should be considered if a transthoracic study is not confirmatory, if the patient presents with a stroke, or if ASD closure is considered.

Consider cardiac catheterization
Measurement of oxygen saturation in the right atrium, RV, and PA allows confirmation of the shunt and quantification of its size.
Formal evaluation of pulmonary hypertension can be performed.

Perform serial examinations in patients with small ASDs
Many ASDs identified in infancy will close spontaneously by the age of 5 years.
Small ASDs (Qp:Qs <1.5:1) identified in adults rarely progress.
- Consider repeat echocardiography every 2 years to assess RV size and function.
Antibiotic prophylaxis is NOT required for patients with ASDs.
- The absence of turbulent flow across ASDs results in a very low risk of subacute bacterial endocarditis.

Consider ASD closure for large shunts
Large shunts identified in childhood should be closed to prevent the development of pulmonary hypertension and RV failure.
ASDs in adults with Qp:Qs >1.5:1, if progressive RV enlargement or RV failure occurs, or the patient develops a stroke.
- Ostium secundum defects may be closed percutaneously using "umbrella" or "clam shell" devices.
  - Requires a rim of tissue (at least 2 m) around the ASD site onto which the device can be implanted.
- Surgical closure should be considered if percutaneous closure is not possible.

Avoid closure of ASDs that are associated with severe pulmonary hypertension and right-to-left shunting (Eisenmenger's syndrome)
Closure of the shunt in this setting results in progressive RV failure.

S

How was the diagnosis made?

Patients most often present with symptoms of significant aortic valve stenosis (AS):

- Dyspnea   • Angina   • Syncope

Less frequently, patients present with symptoms of aortic insufficiency (AI) (predominantly congestive heart failure [CHF]).

Occasionally patients may be asymptomatic and a bicuspid valve is suspected on physical examination or noted incidentally on echocardiography.

How old is the patient?

Symptoms of AS frequently occur at a younger age (fifth or sixth decade) than that expected with acquired disease of a congenitally normal valve.

- The turbulent nature of blood flow across a bicuspid valve predisposes it to earlier fibrocalcific disease.

Patients presenting with AI tend to be in an even younger age group (third or fourth decade of life).

Does the patient have other congenital disorders?

Bicuspid aortic valve (AV) is often associated with aortic coarctation.

- ~10% of patients with a bicuspid AV have aortic coarctation.
- ~50% of patients with aortic coarctation have a bicuspid AV.

Other congenital abnormalities associated with bicuspid AV include:

- Patent ductus arteriosus.
- Turner's syndrome.

Obtain a thorough review of symptoms

Check vital signs

A narrow pulse pressure may be sign of significant valvular stenosis.

A widened pulse pressure may indicate significant valvular insufficiency.

Perform a cardiac examination, looking for

An early systolic ejection click (common with this condition).

Findings consistent with AS. (See SOAP 24.)

- A systolic ejection murmur.
  - The murmur may be late peaking if the valve is severely stenotic.
- A soft or paradoxically split second heart sound.

A murmur of aortic regurgitation. (See SOAP 26.)

- A decrescendo diastolic murmur.

Perform a vascular examination

A delay between the left and right radial pluses or between the radial and femoral pulses is suggestive of concomitant aortic coarctation.

Diminished and slow rising carotid pulses (*pulsus parvus et tardus*) are suggestive of severe aortic stenosis.

Assess for peripheral manifestations of AI. (See SOAP 26.)

Bicuspid aortic valve
Most common form of congenital valvular heart disease. Occurs in 1% to 2% of the general population.
Often develops stenosis or regurgitation between the third and fifth decades of life.
Associated with ascending aortic aneurysm and aortic dissection owing to an inherent aortic abnormality or concomitant aortic coarctation.

Differential diagnosis
- Senile calcific aortic valvular disease
- Subvalvular AS
- Rheumatic heart disease
- Hypertrophic cardiomyopathy

 Obtain an electrocardiogram
Left ventricular hypertrophy and left atrial enlargement may be present with AS or AI.
PR prolongation or heart block may be present.
- Calcification around the AV node can lead to conduction abnormalities.

Obtain a chest radiograph
Dilation of the proximal aorta is common.
Rib notching combined with proximal aortic dilation is suggestive of concomitant aortic coarctation.
Cardiomegaly and pulmonary edema may be present with severe valve dysfunction.

Obtain an echocardiogram
Can usually suggest or confirm the presence of a bicuspid valve.
- Transesophageal echocardiography may further clarify the valve structure if unclear on a transthoracic study.
Can determine the severity of resulting valvular stenosis or regurgitation.
Can assess for associated abnormalities (i.e., aortic coarctation, aortic aneurysm).
Can assess LV size and function.

Refer to cardiology for assistance in managing patients with mild-to-moderate valvular dysfunction
Serial clinical evaluations to assess for the development of symptoms.
Echocardiogram every 2 years in patients with mild AS or mild AI.
Echocardiogram every 6–12 months in patient with moderate to severe AS or AI.

Consider aortic valve replacement in patients with a bicuspid aortic valve in whom there is
Asymptomatic but severe valvular stenosis (AV area <0.8 cm^2) or regurgitation.
Moderate or severe AS or AI with associated symptoms (angina, CHF, or syncope).
Bacterial aortic valve endocarditis.
Progressive aortic dilation.

Prescribe antibiotic prophylaxis for all patients with bicuspid aortic valves, irrespective of valvular dysfunction

S   What are the patient's current symptoms?

Many patients with pulmonary stenosis (PS) are asymptomatic.

Early symptoms include dyspnea on exertion, easy fatigability, and chest pain.

Late symptoms relate to right heart failure (ascites, peripheral edema).

Exertional syncope may also occur.

Does the patient have other congenital cardiac abnormalities?

Valvular PS is usually an isolated cardiac abnormality.

- May occur with ventricular septal defect (VSD) or subvalvular PS, or as part of Noonan's syndrome.
  - Noonan's syndrome: webbed neck, low-set ears, hypertelorism, valvular PS.

Subvalvular PS is usually associated with a VSD, or as part of tetrology of Fallot.

Supravalvular PS is often associated with other cardiac anomalies.

- Atrial septal defect (ASD), VSD, valvular PS, Tetralogy of Fallot, William's syndrome.
  - Williams syndrome: infantile hypercalcemia, elfin facies, mental retardation, and supravalvular pulmonary stenosis.

Obtain a medical history

Congenital rubella infection is associated with supravalvular PS.

Obtain a family history

Occasionally, supravalvular PS (and rarely valvular PS) may be familial.

O   Check vital signs

Decreased oxygen saturation may indicate the presence of shunting across an associated atrial or ventricular septal defect.

Perform a physical examination, looking for the following features

Characteristic features of William's or Noonan's syndrome.

Cyanosis and digital clubbing are associated with intracardiac shunts.

Jugular venous pressure is usually elevated, often with a prominent 'v' wave from tricuspid regurgitation.

A systolic thrill may be palpable over the left second and third interspaces.

A right ventricular heave may be felt along the left sternal border.

The second heart sound is widely split with a soft and delayed pulmonic component (P_2).

A harsh crescendo-decrescendo murmur is usually heard along the left sternal border.

- Louder upon inspiration.
- May be associated with an early systolic ejection click.

Obtain an electrocardiogram

Right ventricular hypertrophy (right axis deviation with RsR' in lead V_1) and right atrial enlargement are usually present.

Obtain a chest radiograph

Post-stenotic dilation of the pulmonary arteries.

Diminution of pulmonary vascular markings.

Right ventricular enlargement.

Pulmonary stenosis
Structural narrowing of the pulmonary valve resulting in pressure overload of the right ventricle. It is primarily a congenital disorder; usually an isolated finding but may occur with other cardiac abnormalities. Can be classified into obstruction at the valvular level (90% of cases), at the subvalvular level, or at the supravalvular level.
Factors associated with valvular stenosis:

- Isolated congenital abnormality
- Noonan's syndrome
- Carcinoid disease

- Rheumatic disease rarely if ever effects the pulmonary valve.

Factors associated with subvalvular stenosis:
- Tetralogy of Fallot (classically pulmonary infundibular stenosis).

Factors associated with supravalvular stenosis:
- Congenital Rubella syndrome (pulmonary arterial stenosis).
- Williams syndrome.

Classification of severity of PS
Normal pulmonary valve (PV): area 2.0 cm^2/m^2 of body surface area and no transvalvular gradient.
Mild PS: valve area >1.0 cm^2/m^2, peak pressure gradient <50 mm Hg.
Moderate PS: valve area 0.5 to 1.0 cm^2/m^2, peak pressure gradient 50 to 80 mm Hg.
Severe PS: valve area <0.5 cm^2/m^2, peak pressure gradient >80 mm Hg.

 Obtain an echocardiogram
Can confirm the diagnosis, assess severity of PS, quantify RV size and function, and identify other congenital abnormalities.
Can define the site of obstruction (sub-, supra-, or valvular) and estimate transvalvular gradient.

Consider right and left heart catheterization
Rarely necessary: usually reserved for patients in whom the diagnosis is uncertain or in whom surgical or percutaneous valvuloplasty is being considered.
Gold standard for defining right ventricular pressure and the gradient across the PV.
Can identify and quantify associated intracardiac shunts.

Institute medical therapy
Diuretics as needed to control symptoms of right heart failure.
Antibiotic prophylaxis for infective endocarditis.

Consider surgical options depending on the nature and severity of stenosis
Mild PS (valvular or nonvalvular):
- Does not require correction: 94% survival at 20 years after diagnosis.

Moderate valvular PS:
- Conservative therapy in asymptomatic patients with normal RV function.
- Consider balloon valvuloplasty in patients with symptoms or RV dysfunction.

Severe valvular PS:
- Percutaneous balloon valvuloplasty, even in asymptomatic patients.
  - 60% of patients will develop symptoms or RV failure within 10 years.
- Surgery if valvuloplasty not possible.

Moderate to severe nonvalvular PS:
- Surgical correction in symptomatic patients, if technically feasible.

S **Does the patient have any cardiovascular symptoms (chest pain or heart failure)?**

Patients with Marfan syndrome are prone to aortic aneurysm and dissection.

- The pain of aortic dissection is often a severe, tearing pain that radiates to the interscapular region.

Aortic root dilation may cause aortic insufficiency and result in congestive heart failure (CHF).

Associated mitral valve prolapse and regurgitation may cause palpitations or symptoms of CHF.

Pleuritic chest pain, especially with shortness of breath, may suggest spontaneous pneumothorax.

Does the patient have any musculoskeletal symptoms?

Scoliosis or kyphosis may cause back pain.

Patients may note hypermobility of their joints.

Does patient have any abnormal visual/ocular conditions?

- Myopia	- Retinal detachment	- Retinal tears
- Glaucoma	- Iritis	- Proliferative retinopathy

- 50% to 80% of Marfan patients have *ectopia lentis* (upward lens displacement)

Is there a family history of Marfan syndrome?

70% of cases are hereditary in an autosomal dominant pattern; the remainder are sporadic.

O **Review vital signs**

A widened pulse pressure may indicate aortic insufficiency.

Perform a focused physical examination looking for signs of Marfan syndrome

Tall, thin body habitus.

Arm span exceeding height (arm span to height ratio >1.05).

Reduced upper to lower body ratio (<0.85 vs. 0.93 in normal).

Arachnodactyly of fingers and toes.

"Thumb sign:" When the thumb is enclosed in a clenched fist, the distal portion of the thumb extends beyond the border of the hand.

"Wrist sign:" When grasping the wrist, the first and fifth digits touch.

Pectus excavatum or carinatum, scoliosis, spondylolisthesis, or high arched palate

Perform a cardiac and vascular examination

Examine for peripheral signs of aortic insufficiency. (See SOAP 26.)

Listen for the murmur of aortic regurgitation, mitral valve prolapse, or mitral regurgitation.

A **Marfan syndrome**

An inherited condition that is almost always the result of a mutation of the fibrillin 1 gene on chromosome 15, which encodes for fibrillin, an important component of elastic tissues. Related gene mutations (TGF-β receptor-2) may produce a Marfan phenotype.

Diagnostic criteria

Must have involvement of at least three of the following systems:

- Skeletal (pectus carinatum, scoliosis, wrist and thumb signs, arm span:height ratio >1.05).
- Ocular (lens dislocation).
- Cardiovascular (aortic dilation, aortic dissection, mitral valve prolapse).

- Dura (lumbosacral dural ectasia on computed tomography or magnetic resonance imaging).
- Genetic (first-degree relative with Marfan syndrome, fibrillin 1 mutation on genetic testing).

Differential diagnosis
Homocystinuria may mimic Marfan syndrome.
MASS syndrome: Mitral valve prolapse, Aortic root mildly dilated, Skin abnormalities (stretch marks), and Skeletal features.
- Not associated with progression to aneurysm or risk of dissection.
Ehlers-Danlos syndrome: joint hypermobility +/− mitral valve prolapse.

P

Initiate prophylactic beta-blocker therapy in all patients
Slows the rate of aortic dilation.
Titrate dose so that heart rate during submaximal exercise is <110 bpm.
Verapamil or diltiazem can be used in patients who are intolerant of beta-blockers.

Discuss exercise limitations with the patient
Avoid high intensity exercise (running, competitive team sports), bursts of exercise (sprinting), or exercises that significantly raise blood pressure (weightlifting).

Obtain ophthalmologic evaluation
For assessment of visual acuity, ectopia lentis, retinal detachment.

Consider computed tomography or magnetic resonance imaging of lumbar spine
To evaluate for dural ectasia (a major finding of Marfan syndrome) if its presence would clinch the diagnosis.

Obtain serial echocardiography to measure the aortic root size
If aortic root diameter <45 mm, screen with echocardiography yearly.
If aortic root diameter >45 mm, screen every 6 months.

Consider elective aortic root replacement when the aortic root diameter is >50 mm
Elective repair is associated with lower mortality than is emergent repair.

Provide preconception counseling for all women with Marfan syndrome
The risk of aortic dissection increases significantly during pregnancy.
The risk of transmission from the affected mother to the child is 50%.

Provide endocarditis prophylaxis for patients with aortic insufficiency

If symptomatic, evaluate for surgical repair of severe pectus excavatum or scoliosis

Consider screening family members
Examination may identify classic phenotypic findings.
Genetic tests can identify the mutant gene.

S **What are the patient's symptoms?**

Many patients with congenital heart disease (CHD) are asymptomatic. When present, symptoms depend on the specific malformation and the cardiac chambers involved, and may include:

- Dyspnea
- Orthopnea
- Paroxysmal nocturnal dyspnea
- Pedal edema
- Cyanosis
- Fatigue
- Syncope
- Palpitations

Obtain a medical history

Did the patient have a murmur in childhood?

Has the patient had corrective cardiac surgery?

Is there a family history of congenital heart disease?

Was the patient exposed to toxins in utero?

Lithium: associated with Ebstein's anomaly.

Alcohol: associated with ventricular septal defect (VSD).

Dilantin: associated with pulmonary stenosis, aortic stenosis, patent ductus arteriosus (PDA), and aortic coarctation.

Rubella: associated with atrial septal defect (ASD), PDA, pulmonary valvular or arterial stenosis.

Obtain a thorough review of systems

As a child, was the patient able to "keep up with" other children?

Has the patient ever had cyanotic episodes?

Has the patient had symptoms of left or right heart failure?

O **Identify classic features of congenital syndromes with cardiac manifestations**

Turner's syndrome: short female with webbed neck and low-set ears.

- Associated with aortic coarctation, bicuspid aortic valve.

Down's syndrome: hypotonia, prominent occiput, micrognathia, single palmar crease.

- Associated with endocardial Cushing defects, ASD, VSD.

Holt-Oram: skeletal abnormalities of upper extremities, clavicular hypoplasia.

- Associated with ASD.

Williams: elfin facies, mental deficiency.

- Associated with supravalvar aortic and pulmonic stenosis.

Central cyanosis suggests an ASD or VSD with right-to-left shunting of blood.

Check vital signs including the oxygen saturation

Low oxygen saturations may indicate the presence of right-to-left shunting.

A difference in left and right arm blood pressures suggests an aortic coarctation.

Perform a cardiac examination, looking for

Jugular venous pressure: increased in patients with right ventricular (RV) failure or tricuspid regurgitation (i.e., Ebstein's anomaly).

Displaced point of maximal impulse: will be on the right side of the chest with dextrocardia.

Right ventricular heave: suggests RV pressure/volume overload (ASD, VSD, PS).

Listen for the murmur of:

- Aortic stenosis: harsh systolic murmur at right upper sternal border.
- Pulmonic stenosis: harsh systolic murmur at left upper sternal border.
- ASD: pulmonary ejection murmur at left upper sternal border.
- VSD: holosystolic murmur at left sternal border.
- PDA: continuous murmur at left upper sternal border.

A **Congenital heart disease**

Congenital abnormalities in the development of the heart leading to intracardiac shunting, abnormal valvular function, ventricular pressure or volume overload, and/or ventricular failure.

Most frequent abnormalities

- Bicuspid aortic valve (see SOAP 31)
- VSD (see SOAP 29)
- PDA
- Marfan syndrome (see SOAP 33)
- Mitral valve prolapse
- ASD (see SOAP 30)
- Aortic coarctation (see SOAP 50)
- Pulmonic stenosis (see SOAP 32)
- Eisenmenger's: ASD, VSD, or PDA with pulmonary hypertension and right-to-left shunt
- Tetralogy of Fallot: VSD, overriding aorta, pulmonary outflow obstruction, right ventricular hypertrophy
- Ebstein's anomaly: apical displacement of the tricuspid valve into the RV with severe TR
  - 50% have an ASD or patent foramen ovale; 25% have at least one bypass tract (Wolff-Parkinson-White syndrome)
- Kartagener syndrome: dextrocardia with sinusitis, situs inversus, bronchiectasis

P

Obtain an electrocardiogram

Look for evidence of atrial or ventricular enlargement, and conduction problems.
Reverse R wave progression (tall R wave in lead V_1 with progressively decreased amplitude across the precordium) suggests dextrocardia.

Obtain a chest radiograph

ASD or VSD: dilated RV, right atrium (RA), and pulmonary artery (PA); increased pulmonary vascularity.
Eisenmenger's: dilated RV, RA, and PA; pruning of peripheral pulmonary vessels.
Aortic coarctation: aortic "figure-3" sign, notching of inferior rib margins.
Ebstein's: marked RA dilation, small PA.
Dextrocardia: heart is in right hemithorax; gastric bubble on right (situs inversus).

Obtain noninvasive imaging study to define cardiac anatomy in patients with suspected CHD

Transthoracic echocardiogram (TTE): usually the initial test of choice.
  - Can assess valvular abnormalities, identify and quantify shunts, assess LV and RV function, and estimate PA pressure.
Transesophageal echocardiogram: useful in identifying shunts not seen on TTE.
Cardiac magnetic resonance imaging.
  - May define complex anatomic abnormalities better than echocardiography.
  - Can assess associated abnormalities of the coronary arteries and the aorta.
  - Can assess, identify, and quantify shunts.

Consult cardiology to help determine further evaluation and management

Consider cardiac catheterization

Provides further data on cardiac function and structure; reveals coronary anatomy.
Can accurately assess pulmonary pressure and quantify shunts.

Consider percutaneous or surgical closure of shunts (ASD, VSD, PDA)

Consider closure of all PDAs, ASDs if shunt >1.5 to 2.0:1, VSDs if shunt >2:1.
Patients with Eisenmenger's syndrome are not candidates for shunt closure.
  - The only effective therapy is heart-lung transplantation.

Refer all patients with complex CHD to a facility that specializes in their care

All patients with CHD should receive antibiotic prophylaxis for procedures

Not necessary in patients with isolated ASD or corrected shunts.

S
How was the diagnosis made?
Patients with first-degree atrioventricular block (AVB) are usually asymptomatic
The diagnosis is made on an electrocardiogram (ECG).
- A PR interval of >200 msec on an ECG is diagnostic.

First-degree AVB occurring with other conduction abnormalities may be a cause of
symptoms (e.g., syncope or presyncope).

Does the patient have factors that predispose to a first-degree AVB?
Medications: β-blockers, calcium channel blockers, digoxin.
Sclerocalcific disease of the AV node.
- Degenerative process associated with increasing age.
- Degeneration accelerated with renal failure.

Prior valve replacement surgery.
Electrolyte disturbance: hyperkalemia, hypocalcemia.
Ischemia (especially inferior myocardial infarction).
Hypothyroidism.
Rheumatic fever.

Does the patient have a prior history of syncope?
Syncope in the setting of a first-degree AVB may indicate intermittent higher degree
AVB.

Perform a review of systems
Evaluate for symptoms of cardiac disease, especially presyncope or syncope.
May detect symptoms of hypothyroidism.

Perform a physical examination
Bradycardia suggests suppression of the conduction system by medications.
Cardiac examination may reveal the murmur of aortic stenosis, suggesting degenerative/
calcific disease of the conduction system.
Examination is frequently normal.

Review the patient's ECG
Essential for diagnosis: PR interval is >200 ms.
May reveal other conduction abnormalities (e.g., bundle branch block (BBB) or axis
deviation).
- First-degree AVB in the presence of a BBB usually indicates disease of the His-
Purkinje system, not the AV node.
- First-degree AVB with bifascicular block (either a right BBB and left anterior
fascicular block, or a left BBB), indicates disease of the one remaining fascicle
(i.e., trifascicular block) and may be an indication for permanent pacemaker
placement.

Review electrolytes and thyroid function tests

First-Degree atrioventricular heart block
A delay in the propagation of electrical depolarization from the atrium to the ventricles. Manifests as a prolongation of the PR interval on the ECG (PR interval >200 msec).

Pathophysiology
AV conduction may be slowed owing to the effects of medications or increased vagal tone on the AV node, or may reflect true disease of the conduction system.

Compare current electrocardiogram to a previous tracing
Stability of the R interval is reassuring.
Progressive prolongation of the PR interval over time suggests worsening conduction system disease.

Review medication list
Consider stopping AV nodal medications in patients with very prolonged PR interval (>250 msec) or in any patient with presyncope or syncope.

Reassure the patient
In the absence of underlying heart disease, this is a benign condition.
In the absence of symptoms it is usually not necessary to do anything specifically to treat a first-degree AVB aside from correcting possible causes.

Consider obtaining an exercise test
Not necessary in most asymptomatic patients.
Consider in patients in whom symptoms suggest higher degree of AV block.
* Patients with intrinsic disease of the conduction system often develop higher degree of AVB at higher heart rates during exercise.
* Patients with first-degree AVB from increased vagal tone or medications will often have a shorter PR interval at higher heart rates as a result of exercise-induced withdrawal of vagal tone.

Consider obtaining an echocardiogram
Not necessary in the absence of symptoms or physical findings suggestive of underlying heart disease.
May be useful in patients with:
* Symptoms (to rule out structural heart disease).
* A murmur on physical examination.

Treat other reversible causes of 1st degree AVB
Correct electrolyte disturbances.
Treat hypothyroidism with replacement therapy.

S **How did the patient present?**
Most patients are asymptomatic; the diagnosis is made incidentally on electrocardiogramy (ECG).
Occasionally patients may present with the following symptoms:
- Lightheadedness, dizziness
- Presyncope or syncope
- Orthostasis
- Palpitations

Does the patient have predisposing factors for heart block?
Medications: atrioventricular (AV) nodal blocking agents (e.g., β-blockers, calcium channel blockers, digoxin).
Advanced age.
Infection (e.g., endocarditis with valvular ring abscess; Lyme disease).
Electrolyte disturbances (e.g., hyperkalemia, hypocalcemia).
Ischemia (especially post-myocardial infarction).
Cardiac surgery.
High vagal tone.

O **Check vital signs**
Second-degree heart block is often associated with bradycardia.
- Results from effects of medications or high vagal tone.
Hypotension is unusual except with marked bradycardia.
Hypertension may paradoxically be present due to a reflexive excess of sympathetic tone.

Perform a physical examination
Is frequently unremarkable.
Observe the jugular venous pressure:
- Cannon "a" waves may be seen with intermittent non conducted atrial contractions. These occur when the atrium contracts against a closed tricuspid valve.

Review the patient's electrocardiogram
Carefully decipher the relationship between P waves and the QRS complexes.
A long rhythm strip may be necessary to make the diagnosis.
Look for evidence of ischemia or infarction.
Look for other conduction system disease (e.g., bundle branch block).

Review electrolytes and renal function tests
Renal dysfunction predisposes to electrolyte abnormalities (i.e., hyperkalemia).

Consider obtaining an echocardiogram if the history and examination suggest structural heart disease
May reveal aortic or mitral valve disease or evidence of ischemia/infarction.

Second-degree atrioventricular heart block
Refers to the intermittent loss of AV conduction. Manifests on ECG as an intermittent appropriately timed P wave without a subsequent QRS complex (a "dropped beat").

Classification
Mobitz type I (also called "Wenckebach"):
- Gradual prolongation of the PR interval until a dropped beat occurs.
- Characterized by "group beating" (recurring pattern) on a rhythm strip.
- Usually the result of increased vagal tone or medications.
- Occurs at slower heart rates.
- Usually a benign rhythm that does not progress to more severe heart block (HB).

Mobitz type II:
- Dropped beats occur without preceding PR segment prolongation.
- Usually reflects structural disease of the conduction system.
- Occurs at higher heart rates.
- Frequently progresses to more severe AV block (i.e., CHB).

Differential diagnosis
Sinus rhythm with blocked premature atrial complexes (PAC).
- PACs may be blocked if they occur when the AV node is refractory.

Course atrial fibrillation.
Atrial flutter with variable block.
Complete heart block.

Review ECG carefully to determine the type of second-degree HB that is present

Consult cardiology if the diagnosis is unclear and for all patients with Mobitz II HB

Admit symptomatic patients to a monitored setting
Asymptomatic patients with Wenckebach can be reassured.
Asymptomatic patients with Mobitz II HB may also need monitoring.

Treat reversible causes
Correct electrolyte imbalances if present.
Decrease or discontinue all AV nodal blocking agents, if possible.
Treat ischemia if present.

Institute specific therapy based on symptoms and the type of HB present
Mobitz type I:
- Treat symptomatic patients with atropine (0.05 mg IV up to 0.3 mg).
  - Consider IV glucagon for β-blocker toxicity and IV calcium for calcium channel blocker toxicity.
- Rarely requires a temporary or permanent pacemaker.

Mobitz type II:
- If asymptomatic, close follow-up is required as a proportion proceed to complete heart block over the next year if left untreated.
  - Consider Holter monitoring to exclude intermittent higher degree AV block.
  - Consider obtaining an exercise test: Patients with Mobitz II HB will frequently develop worsened HB at faster heart rates.
- Refer for placement of a permanent pacemaker if symptomatic or with persistent Mobitz II HB after an MI.

S **What are the patient's symptoms?**
Common presenting symptoms include:
- Palpitations
- Dyspnea on exertion
- Fatigue/lethargy
- Presyncope or syncope
  - ◆ May result from marked bradycardia or from the development of bradycardia-induced polymorphic ventricular tachycardia.

Does the patient have predisposing factors?
Medications: atrioventricular (AV) nodal blocking agents (e.g., β-blockers, calcium channel blockers, digoxin).
Infiltrative disorders: amyloidosis, sarcoidosis, hemochromatosis.
Infection: Lyme disease.
Electrolyte disturbance: hyperkalemia, hypocalcemia.
Ischemia (especially after an inferior myocardial infarction).
Hypothyroidism.
Prior cardiac surgery (especially after aortic valve replacement).

Review medications
Identify all AV nodal blocking agents.
Identify medications that cause electrolyte abnormalities (e.g., angiotensin-converting enzyme inhibitors, angiotensin receptor blockers, diuretics).

Perform a review of systems and a social/travel history
May elicit symptoms of previously undetected thyroid dysfunction.
Recent outdoor activities in endemic areas: Consider Lyme disease.
Travel to rural South America: Consider Chagas disease.

O **Check vital signs**
Hypotension and marked bradycardia are indications for pacing for complete heart block (CHB).
Marked bradycardia is often associated with a widened pulse pressure.

Perform a physical examination
Observe the jugular venous pulse for prominent A waves (*cannon "a" waves*).
- Occur when the atrium contracts against a closed tricuspid valve.
- Cannon A waves are pathognomonic of AV dissociation.
Cardiac auscultation may reveal variable intensity of the heart sounds.
Assess for evidence of pulmonary congestion.
Look for evidence of poor perfusion (confusion, cool extremities, etc).
Perform a cranial nerve exam and search for the rash of Lyme disease.

Review the patient's electrocardiogram
Diagnostic features of CHB:
- P waves have no relationship to the QRS complexes (AV dissociation).
- The atrial rate exceeds that of the ventricles.
The width of the QRS complex reflects the site of the escape rhythm.
- Junctional escape rhythms generally have a narrow QRS complex.
  - ◆ Usually hemodynamically stable.
- Ventricular escape rhythms are associated with wide QRS complexes.
  - ◆ Usually very unstable rhythms and warrant the emergent use of transcutaneous or transvenous pacing.

Complete heart block
Refers to the complete inability of atrial impulses to conduct to the ventricles. May result from disease of the AV node or the infranodal conduction system. Results in the atria and ventricles beating independently of each other and manifests on ECG as dissociation of the P waves and QRS complexes (AV dissociation).

Etiology
Structural disease of the conduction system.
* Infection, infarction, infiltration, or degenerative diseases.

Functional abnormality of the conduction system.
* AV nodal blocking medications or increased vagal tone.

Differential diagnosis
Ventricular tachycardia, accelerated idioventricular rhythm, and accelerated junctional rhythms.
* AV dissociation is present in all these rhythms. They differ from CHB in that the atrial rate is slower than the ventricular rate.

Institute temporary pacing
May be performed transcutaneously or transvenously.

Transcutaneous pacing is performed via pads placed on the chest.
* May be painful and requires sedation.

Transvenous pacers are inserted into the RV via a central venous catheter.
* Consists of a balloon-tipped catheter with electrodes on its tip.
* Can be placed with ECG guidance or with fluoroscopy.
* Pacing threshold should be <1 mv and the pacing output should be set at three times the pacing threshold as a safety margin.

Admit to the intensive care unit and obtain a cardiology consult

Identify and treat reversible causes of CHB
Correct electrolyte abnormalities and obtain thyroid function tests.

Decrease or discontinue all AV nodal blocking agents.

Treat ischemia if present.

Administer atropine (0.05 mg IV, up to 0.3 mg) if suspect functional HB.
* Dopamine is useful in patients with associated hypotension or congestive heart failure.

Administer IV glucagon for β-blocker toxicity and IV calcium for calcium channel blocker toxicity.

Obtain a stat digoxin level in patients taking this medication.
* Toxicity is common at levels >2.0 ng/mL (may occur at >1.0 ng/mL).
* Give digoxin-specific antibodies if CHB results from digoxin toxicity.
  * Number of vials of antibody = [digoxin level × wt in kg]/100.

Check Lyme titers and treat if consistent with infection.

Obtain an echocardiogram
May suggest possible etiologies of the arrhythmia.

Patients with left ventricular ejection fraction <30% may need an implantable cardiac defibrillator as well as a pacemaker.

Consider implantation of a permanent pacemaker
All patients with irreversible CHB require permanent pacemaker insertion.

Pacing leads are inserted into the right atrium and right ventricle (RV) to maintain AV synchrony (in only atrial fibrillation a RV lead is used).

S **What are the patient's symptoms?**
Patients with wide complex tachycardia (WCT) may present with a wide variety of
symptoms, including:
- Palpitations
- Lightheadedness
- Angina
- Dyspnea
- Presyncope
- Shock
- Diaphoresis
- Syncope
- Hemodynamic instability

The presence or absence of symptoms does not help differentiate supraventricular
tachycardia (SVT) from ventricular tachycardia (VT).

Does the patient have a history of arrhythmias?
If so, the WCT is often the same as the prior arrhythmia.

Does the patient have a history of structural heart disease?
A WCT in a patient with a history of cardiac disease, especially ischemic heart disease, is much more likely to be VT than SVT.

**Does the patient have a permanent pacemaker or implantable cardiac
defibrillator (ICD)?**
These devices can predispose to development of device-mediated tachycardia.
The presence of an ICD suggests that the patient is at risk for VT.

Is the patient on medications that predispose to arrhythmias?
Several medications can prolong the QT interval and result in polymorphic VT.
Antiarrhythmic agents (quinidine, procainamide, sotalol, disopyramide).
Antimicrobial agents (erythromycin, pentamidine, quinolones).
Antipsychotic agents (chlorpromazine, haloperidol, thioridazine).

O **Check the vital signs**
Hypotension is common during WCTs and mandates urgent therapy.

Perform a cardiac examination looking especially for
Jugular venous pulse: presence of cannon "a" waves during a WCT suggests atrioven-
tricular (AV) dissociation and is diagnostic of VT.
- Cannon "a" waves are prominent pulsations in the JVP resulting from atrial
contraction against a closed tricuspid valve.
Heart sounds: Variable intensity of S_1 is also suggestive of AV dissociation.

Review the chest radiograph looking for evidence of
   - Cardiomegaly   - Prior cardiac surgery   - Pacemaker or ICD

Review the patient's 12-lead electrocardiogram
Features that suggest a WCT is VT include:
- AV dissociation (the P waves are unrelated to the QRS complexes).
- Capture or fusion beats. (See SOAP 44.)
- A shift in QRS axis when compared to the patient's baseline ECG.
- An extreme right axis deviation (axis: –90 to –180 degrees).
- QRS width of >160 ms.
If the QRS morphology during a WCT is identical to the patient's baseline ECG, or
is characteristic of a normal left bundle branch block (BBB) or right BBB, the
rhythm is likely an SVT.

Request an electrolyte panel
Abnormalities of potassium, magnesium, and calcium can precipitate WCT.

Wide complex tachycardia
Defined as HR >100 beats/min with a QRS width >120 ms (3 small boxes on an electrocardiogram [ECG]).

Differential diagnosis
- Ventricular tachycardia   - SVT with rate-related aberrancy
- SVT with a baseline wide QRS complex (e.g., left BBB, paced rhythm)
- Pacemaker mediated tachycardia

It is essential to determine whether a WCT is VT or SVT—misdiagnosis of VT as SVT can lead to detrimental consequences if improper therapy is used.

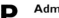 **Admit to a monitored setting**

Use the history, examination, and ECG to differentiate VT from SVT with aberrancy
If unable to determine the nature of a WCT, it should be treated as VT.

Perform immediate electrical defibrillation of hemodynamically unstable patients
Start at 100 J of energy and increase to 200 to 360 J if necessary.

Institute pharmacologic therapy and attempt abortive maneuvers in stable patients
If there is no doubt that the rhythm is SVT:
- Attempt to abort with vagal maneuvers (carotid sinus massage, Valsalva).
- IV adenosine (6-mg bolus followed by a 12-mg bolus if needed) is highly effective in terminating SVT and has a short half-life (6 seconds).
If the patient is stable and there is no doubt that the rhythm is VT:
- Start intravenous lidocaine or amiodarone.
If the patient is hemodynamically stable and the rhythm is uncertain:
- Consider performing carotid sinus massage (CSM):
  - Certain SVTs (AVNRT or AVRT) may terminate with CSM.
  - Sinus tachycardia will slow transiently with CSM.
  - VT is generally unresponsive to CSM.

  - CSM should not be performed in patients with carotid bruits or prior history of cerebrovascular disease.

- Consider empiric use of IV amiodarone, procainamide, or lidocaine.
  - Amiodarone and procainamide are effective for both SVT and VT.
  - Lidocaine is effective for VT but not SVT.

Identify and treat any predisposing factors
Discontinue medications that may prolong the QT interval.
Correct electrolyte abnormalities.

Obtain an echocardiogram
To evaluate LVEF and assess for evidence of prior MI.

Obtain a cardiology consult
Assist with distinguishing VT from SVT.
- May require EP study if unable to distinguish on 12-lead ECG.
Determine further diagnostic evaluation and appropriate treatment.
- Consider antiarrhythmic therapy
  - Beta-blockers, verapamil, or amiodarone for SVT.
  - Amiodarone for VT.
- Consider cardiac catheterization for patients with VT and reduced left ventricular ejection fraction.
- Consider EP study and ablation of VT or SVT.
- Consider placement of an ICD in patients with VT.

S **What are the patient's symptoms?**
Palpitations (rapid and irregular) are the most common symptom of atrial
fibrillation (AF).
Other symptoms include chest pain, dyspnea, and stroke.
Abrupt onset of symptoms often correlates with the onset of AF.
  • Timing of symptoms is crucial in defining the duration of AF and guiding
    subsequent management.

Has the patient had previous similar episodes?
AF is often paroxysmal, but may progress to persistent AF over time.

Is the patient able to terminate the symptoms?
Termination of the arrhythmia by vagal maneuvers (Valsalva, cough, carotid sinus
massage) suggests a reentrant arrhythmia (e.g., atrioventricular reentrant tachycardia,
atrioventricular nodal reentry tachycardia) rather than AF.

Does the patient have a known history of heart disease?
Structural heart disease is a common predisposing condition for AF.
Rapid AF can cause demand ischemia in patients with coronary artery disease and
may precipitate congestive heart failure (CHF) in patients with valvular heart
disease or cardiomyopathy.
Ischemia from coronary artery disease can lead to CHF with subsequent AF.
  • Ischemia rarely causes AF in the absence of CHF.

Is there a history of predisposing factors?
  - Hypertension   - CHF
  - Hyperthyroidism   - Acute lung disease
  - Valvular heart disease (predominantly aortic and mitral valve disease)
  - Toxins (alcohol, caffeine, cocaine, amphetamines)

Review medications
Is the patient on thyroid replacement, theophylline, or inhaled β-agonists?

O **Review the patient's vital signs**

A rapid and irregularly, irregular pulse is a hallmark of AF.
Hypotension may occur with very fast heart rate (HR) or with underlying heart disease.

Perform a physical examination
S_1 may be of variable intensity; apical HR may exceed perceived radial HR.
Listen carefully for aortic and mitral valve murmurs.
Assess for evidence of heart failure (rales, pleural effusions, elevated JVP).

Review the patent's electrocardiogram
  - Absence of P waves   - An irregularly, irregular ventricular rate

Review laboratory tests
Check electrolytes and thyroid function tests.
Cardiac enzymes should be obtained if there is a clinical suspicion of ischemia based
on the patient's symptoms or ECG.

 Atrial fibrillation
A condition in which multiple competing foci depolarize the atria at rapid rates (400
to 600 beats per minute) resulting in ineffective atrial contraction. The atrial
impulses are filtered by the AV node, resulting in an irregular ventricular rhythm.
Loss of effective atrial contraction predisposes to formation of atrial thrombi, and
may reduce cardiac output and precipitate heart failure, especially in patients with
underlying heart disease.

Differential diagnosis

- Multiple atrial premature contractions
- Multifocal atrial tachycardia
- Atrial flutter with variable block

P **Admit patients with new-onset AF with rapid HR or CHF to a monitored setting**

Control the HR with AV nodal blocking agents (goal HR <100 bpm)
Acutely: IV beta blocker (e.g., metoprolol 5 mg IV) or IV calcium channel blocker (e.g., diltiazem 10 to 20 mg IV).
Consider use of a continuous intravenous diltiazem drip if HR remains high.
Consider use of intravenous digoxin (0.25 mg) for patients with CHF.
Change to oral medication once heart rate control has been achieved.

Anticoagulate to avoid thromboembolism
Initially anticoagulate with heparin and transition to warfarin (goal INR: 2–3).
Anticoagulate all patients with AF lasting >48 hours or of unknown duration.
- Acute onset AF (<48 hours) can be treated with cardioversion without the need for anticoagulation if the time of onset can be clearly defined.
Most patients require lifelong anticoagulation; especially those with:
- Age >65 years
- Hypertension
- Coronary artery disease
- Structural heart disease (left ventricular hypertension, LV dysfunction, valvular heart disease)

Perform emergent electrical cardioversion for hemodynamically unstable patients
Electrically cardiovert with 100 to 360 J of energy.

Review the patient's chest radiograph
Look for signs of cardiac chamber enlargement (RA, LA, or LV) or CHF.

Treat the underlying cause of AF, if identified

Consider elective cardioversion (CV) to reestablish sinus rhythm for stable patients
Can be performed electrically or chemically.
- Pharmacologic cardioversion may be achieved with a single dose of an antiarrhythmic agent (i.e., propafenone, quinidine, or flecainide).
- Consider chronic use of a class III antiarrhythmic agent (e.g., amiodarone or sotalol) to maintain sinus rhythm after initial CV.
Should only be performed after 3 weeks of therapeutic anticoagulation with warfarin (INR >2) or if transesophageal echocardiography reveals no LA thrombus.
Anticoagulation should be continued for at least 3 weeks after cardioversion.
Successful CV does not necessarily decrease the risk of thromboembolism—continue warfarin indefinitely unless the patient is at high risk of bleeding.
Rhythm control or rate control are equivalent approaches in patients who are hemodynamically stable without LV dysfunction.
Cardioversion (CV) may be preferred for patients with CHF who may be dependent on atrial contraction to maintain adequate cardiac output.

Consider obtaining an echocardiogram
If this is the first episode of AF and a recent echo has not been performed, if a murmur is present, or if the AF is complicated by CHF.
- Evaluate left ventricular ejection fraction, valvular function, left ventricular hypertrophy, and chamber sizes.

Consider AF ablation in patients with recurrent episodes or refractory tachycardia

S

What are the patient's symptoms?

Common presenting symptoms include:

- Palpitations
- Dyspnea
- Chest pain
- Fatigue
- Lightheadedness

Less commonly, patients may present with complications of AFL, including:

- Heart failure
- Stroke
- Myocardial infarction

Does the patient have a history of heart disease that predisposes to atrial flutter (AFL)?

- Rheumatic heart disease
- Ischemic heart disease
- Cardiomyopathy
- Atrial or ventricular septal defects
- Mitral or tricuspid valve stenosis or regurgitation

Does the patient have other predisposing conditions?

- Hypertension
- Hyperthyroidism
- Sick sinus syndrome
- Pericarditis
- Chronic obstructive pulmonary disease (COPD)
- Recent cardiac surgery
- Alcohol and other substance abuse (e.g., cocaine, amphetamines, steroids)

Obtain a review of systems

May disclose symptoms suggestive of previous AFL or of hyperthyroidism.

Review medications

Is the patient on thyroid replacement, theophylline, or inhaled β-agonists?

O

Check vital signs

Tachycardia is common.

- The atrial rate in typical flutter is ~300 beats/min. The ventricular rate depends on the degree of AV nodal block: with 2:1 block, the ventricular rate is 150 beats/min; with 3:1 block, it is 100 beats/min, etc.
- A spontaneously slow ventricular rate suggests AV nodal disease.

Hypotension may occur when there is associated structural heart disease (e.g., aortic or mitral stenosis, cardiomyopathy).

Perform a focused physical examination

Look for signs of underlying disorders: goiter (hyperthyroidism), spider nevi (alcoholism), excessive musculature (steroid abuse), wheezes (COPD).

Cardiac examination:

- Variable heart rate may occur due to variable AV conduction. An irregularly irregular rhythm suggests atrial fibrillation. (See SOAP 39.)
- Listen carefully for murmurs.

Review the patient's chest radiograph

Look for cardiomegaly, signs of congestive heart failure, or evidence of COPD.

Review the patient's ECG

Reveals characteristic "flutter waves" occurring at ~300 beats/min.

- Best seen in leads II, III, aVF, V_1; classically have a saw-tooth appearance.
- May not be apparent at fast HR—intravenous adenosine or carotid sinus massage may transiently increase AV nodal block and unmask the flutter waves.

Consider obtaining an echocardiogram

To evaluate for valvular disease in patients with murmurs.

To evaluate ventricular function in patients with associated heart failure.

A transesophageal echocardiograph can be used to evaluate for thrombus in the atria (especially the left atrial appendage) before DC cardioversion.

A **Atrial flutter**
Results from a macro-reentrant circuit in the atrium, typically occurring at a rate of 300 beats per minute.

Classification
Typical atrial flutter (90% of cases): The macro-reentrant circuit (usually counter-clockwise) in the right atrium uses the isthmus between the orifice of the inferior vena cava and the annulus of the tricuspid valve as part of its loop.
Atypical atrial flutter (10% of cases): Does not use the isthmus as part of its loop.

Differential diagnosis
- Course atrial fibrillation
- Multifocal atrial tachycardia
- Atrial tachycardia
- AV nodal reentrant tachycardia

P **Admit patients with new-onset AFL with rapid heart rate (HR) or CHF to a monitored setting**

Correct any identifiable causes of the rhythm disturbance
Check thyroid function tests and treat hyperthyroidism.
Check toxic screen if history is suspicious, and stop offending medications.

Control the heart rate with AV nodal blocking agents (goal HR <100 bpm)
Acutely: IV beta-blocker (e.g., metoprolol 5 mg IV) or IV calcium channel blocker (e.g., diltiazem 10 to 20 mg IV).
Consider use of a continuous IV diltiazem drip if HR remains high.
Consider use of IV digoxin (0.25 mg) for patients with heart failure.
Change to oral medication once heart rate control achieved.

Anticoagulate to avoid thromboembolism
Risk of thromboembolic event similar to that with atrial fibrillation.
Anticoagulate all patients with AFL of >48 hours or if unknown duration.
Initially anticoagulate with heparin and transition to warfarin (goal INR: 2–3).
Consider lifelong anticoagulation in patients with chronic or paroxysmal AFL and high risk markers, unless definitive therapy performed (see below):
  • Age >65 years   • Hypertension
  • CAD   • Structural heart disease

Perform emergent electrical cardioversion for hemodynamically unstable patients
Electrically cardiovert with 50 to 360 J of energy.

Consider elective cardioversion (CV) to reestablish sinus rhythm for stable patients
AFL tends to spontaneously revert to sinus rhythm or degenerate to atrial fibrillation.
Electrical CV may result in long-term maintenance of NSR in some patients.
  • Should only be performed after 3 weeks of therapeutic anticoagulation (INR >2) or if transesophageal echocardiography reveals no LA thrombus.
  • Anticoagulation should be continued for at least 3 weeks after CV.
Pharmacologic CV is less successful than with AF.

Consider percutaneous catheter ablation
Uses radiofrequency energy to burn a line of inhibition across the atrial isthmus thereby interrupting the macro-reentrant circuit and preventing recurrent AFL.
This is a first-line treatment for patients who have significant symptoms during AFL or those who want to avoid long-term medication.

S **If the patient has palpitations, what is their pattern?**
Rapid and regular palpitations suggest atrial flutter or atrial tachycardia.
Rapid and irregular palpitations suggest atrial fibrillation.
Slow and forceful palpitations suggest sinus bradycardia.
"Skipped beats" suggest premature complexes or heart block.

Has the patient had presyncope or syncope?
Usually results from prolonged sinus pauses/sinus arrest.

Has the patient had other symptoms attributable to sick sinus syndrome (SSS)?
Patients with SSS may be asymptomatic or can present with symptoms of tachycardia and/or bradycardia, including:
- Fatigue
- Lightheadedness
- Dyspnea
- Increasing angina
- Decreased exercise capacity

Symptoms often evolve over time with periods of asymptomatic bradycardia followed by palpitations and eventually syncope as the disease progresses.

Does the patient have a history of other cardiac disease that is associated with SSS?
Ischemic heart disease (with atherosclerosis of the SA node artery).
Hypertension (>60% of patients with SSS have hypertension).
Congenital heart disease.
Prior cardiac surgery.
Infiltrative heart disease (amyloidosis, hemochromatosis).
Infectious (Lyme disease, Chagas disease, rheumatic fever).

Is the patient on medications that can induce sinus nodal or AV nodal dysfunction?
- Beta-blockers   - Calcium channel blockers   - Digoxin
- Clonidine   - Antiarrhythmic agents   - Lithium

O **Check the vital signs**
Bradycardia is classically seen but may be interspersed with tachycardia.

Perform a physical examination looking especially for
Evidence of structural heart disease (murmurs, an S_3).
Evidence of vascular disease (diminished pulses, vascular bruits).

Review the patient's 12-lead electrocardiogram
Potential findings of SSS include:
- Inappropriate sinus bradycardia.
- Sinus arrest/sinus pauses.
- Alternating patterns of bradycardia and tachycardia, especially AF.
    ◆ "Tachy-brady syndrome" is seen in over 50% of patients with SSS.
- Evidence of concurrent AV nodal block is present in over 50% of cases.
    - Atrial fibrillation with slow ventricular response in the absence of AV nodal blocking medications suggests AV nodal disease and SSS.

Perform carotid sinus massage
If the history suggests carotid sinus hypersensitivity.

CSM should not be performed in patients with carotid bruits or history of cerebrovascular disease.

A **Sick sinus syndrome**
A condition in which the sinoatrial node is dysfunctional, usually as a result of chronic fibrosis of the conduction system. It usually manifests as inappropriate sinus bradycardia, prolonged sinus pauses, or atrial tachyarrhythmias alternating with bradycardia. AV nodal conduction abnormalities are frequently present.

Differential diagnosis
- Carotid sinus sensitivity syndrome   - Medication induced bradyarrhythmias
- Autonomic dysfunction (e.g., excessive vagal tone)

P **Admit symptomatic patients to a monitored setting**
Asymptomatic patients can usually undergo an outpatient evaluation.

Consider ambulatory cardiac monitoring for asymptomatic patients with bradycardia or pauses on electrocardiography, and for patients with symptoms suggestive of SSS
Useful to correlate symptoms with arrhythmias.
Can identify significant arrhythmias even if asymptomatic.
Pauses of >3 seconds (even if asymptomatic) are an indication for a pacemaker.
24-hour Holter monitor is useful for documenting bradycardia, pauses, or tachy-arrhythmias in patients with frequent arrhythmias.
A 30-day event monitor is useful for capturing more infrequent events.

Stop all nonessential drugs that may exacerbate tachy- or bradyarrhythmias

Check serologic tests for causes of reversible sinus node dysfunction
Thyroid function tests.
Lyme titers (if suspected based on history).

Obtain an echocardiogram
Estimate left ventricular ejection fraction.
Evaluate for structural heart disease.

Start anticoagulation with warfarin in all patients with atrial fibrillation or flutter

Obtain a cardiology consult for patients with confirmed SSS

Proceed to placement of a permanent pacemaker
If symptomatic bradycardia without a reversible cause.
If tachy-brady syndrome when medications that are required to control tachycardia result in excessive bradycardia.
If exertional fatigue or dyspnea associated with chronotropic incompetence (failure of heart rate to rise appropriately with exercise).

Consider placing a permanent pacemaker
For asymptomatic patient with a heart rate <30 beats per minute while awake.
For asymptomatic sinus pauses >3 seconds in duration.
For syncope of unexplained origin in a patient with SSS.

S **What are the patient's symptoms?**
Many patients have electrocardiographic (ECG) abnormalities but no symptoms
  (Wolff-Parkinson-White [WPW] pattern).
When present, the most common symptom is palpitations.
  • May be regular and rapid during atrioventricular reentrant tachycardia (AVRT)
    or irregular and rapid (during atrial fibrillation).
Other common symptoms include:
  • Dyspnea   • Chest pain   • Dizziness
  • Lightheadedness   • Presyncope   • Syncope

Does the patient have a history of arrhythmias?
Symptoms of WPW usually start in childhood or adolescence and patients will often
  be aware of the diagnosis.

Is there a family history of arrhythmias?
~3% to 4% of patients with WPW have a family member with the condition.

Does the patient have a history of structural heart disease?
WPW is usually an isolated condition; however, ~10% of patients with Epstein's
  anomaly (see SOAP 27) will have WPW syndrome.

O **Check the vital signs**
Hypotension can occur during AVRT and warrants urgent therapy.

Obtain a 12-lead ECG
May be normal when in normal sinus rhythm (a "concealed bypass tract").
Usually reveals evidence of ventricular pre-excitation:
  • Short PR interval.
  • Slurred onset to a wide QRS complex (the "delta wave").
May reveal one of several tachyarrhythmias:
  • Narrow QRS complex AVRT (orthodromic AVRT – see below).
  • Wide QRS complex AVRT (antidromic AVRT – see below).
  • Atrial fibrillation with very rapid ventricular rate and marked variability in
    QRS width and morphology.
    ◆ 10% to 30% of patients with WPW develop atrial fibrillation.

A **Wolff-Parkinson-White syndrome**
A condition in which an abnormal electrical connection (a *bypass* tract; the Bundle
  of Kent) exists between the atria and ventricles allowing for the rapid conduction
  of electrical impulses from the atria to the ventricles without the usual filtering
  effect of the AV node. Conduction via the bypass tract results in earlier activation
  (preexcitation) of the ventricles than if the impulse had traveled through the AV
  node and predisposes to reentrant arrhythmias using the AV node and the bypass
  tract as the two limbs of the reentrant circuit.
A reentrant loop using the AV node as the antegrade limb and the bypass tract as the
  retrograde limb (orthodromic AVRT) produces a narrow complex tachycardia.
  • Retrograde P waves may be seen after the T waves (long RP tachycardia).
A re-entrant loop using the bypass tract as the antegrade limb and the AV node as
  the retrograde limb (orthodromic AVRT) produces a wide complex tachycardia.

Differential diagnosis
        - Sinus tachycardia   - Atrial flutter
        - AV nodal reentrant tachycardia   - Atrial fibrillation
        - Paroxysmal atrial tachycardia (PAT)

Patients with ECG evidence of a bypass tract but without tachyarrhythmias have *WPW pattern.* Patients with ECG findings and tachyarrhythmias have *WPW syndrome*

P Admit patients with WPW and tachyarrhythmias to a monitored setting

Obtain a cardiology consult
To confirm the diagnosis and assist with acute and chronic management.

Control acute tachyarrhythmias
If the patient is hemodynamically unstable perform immediate electrical defibrillation starting at 100 J of energy.
The treatment for hemodynamically stable patients with AV nodal dependent rhythms (orthodromic or antidromic AVRT) is blockade of the AV node.
- Vagal maneuvers (e.g., carotid sinus massage).
- Adenosine (6 mg IV followed by 12 mg IV if needed).
- Diltiazem (10 to 20 mg IV), Verapamil (5 to 10 mg IV), metoprolol (2.5 to 5 mg IV).
- Antidromic AVRT may look exactly like VT—the above agents should not be given unless it is certain that the rhythm is antidromic AVRT.
  - If uncertain, the rhythm should be treated as VT. (See SOAP 44.)
The treatment of SVTs that are independent of the AV node (atrial fibrillation, atrial flutter, atrial tachycardia) is NOT to block the AV node as this may preferentially shunt conduction down the bypass tract at rapid rates and precipitate hemodynamic collapse.
- Procainamide (50 mg/min IV for 20 minutes) or amiodarone (150 mg/min over 10 minutes followed by a continuous infusion) slow conduction through the bypass tract and may revert the SVT.

Prevent recurrent tachyarrhythmias
Patients with only rare episodes of AVRT can be taught to abort the episodes with vagal maneuvers (e.g., Valsalva maneuver, gagging, etc.).
For patients with frequent recurrences:
- Class Ic antiarrhythmic agents are the first-line pharmacological therapy.
  - Flecainide or propafenone.
- Class III agents (amiodarone, sotalol) may also be effective.
- Chronic administration of AV nodal blocking agents (digoxin, verapamil, diltiazem, or beta-blockers) may also be effective but should be avoided in patients with a history of atrial fibrillation or flutter.

Consider performing radiofrequency ablation
Radiofrequency ablation of the bypass tract provides definitive therapy and is the current standard of care for the long-term prevention of recurrent arrhythmias in this setting.

S **What are the patient's symptoms?**

Patients with atrioventricular nodal reentrant tachycardia (ANVRT) can present
with various symptoms

- Palpitations
- Lightheadedness
- Angina

- Dyspnea
- Presyncope
- Hemodynamic instability

- Chest pain
- Syncope

Was the onset of symptoms gradual or sudden?

The symptoms of AVNRT usually develop suddenly and terminate suddenly.
Symptoms relate to the heart rate and the presence of structural heart disease.

What was the patient doing when the symptoms began?

Often there is no precipitant for AVNRT.
Drugs (nicotine, cocaine, alcohol) and occasionally exercise can initiate it.

O **Check the vital signs**

AVNRT is usually associated with a heart rate of 120–220 beats/minute.
Hypotension can occur with AVNRT and warrants urgent therapy.

Perform a cardiac examination looking especially for

Jugular venous pressure: cannon "A" waves may be present as a result of the simulta-
neous contraction of the atria and ventricles.

- Cannon "a" waves are prominent pulsations in the JVP resulting from atrial
  contraction against a closed tricuspid valve.

Listen for evidence of underlying heart disease (additional heart sounds, murmurs, etc).

Review the chest radiograph, looking for evidence of

    - Cardiomegaly   - Prior cardiac surgery   - Pacemaker or implantable
                                                                cardiac defibrillatory

Obtain a 12-lead electrocardiograph

Features that suggest AVNRT include:

- Narrow complex tachycardia.
- Regular rhythm.
- Absent P waves.
- Inverted P waves in the terminal portion of the QRS in typical AVNRT resulting
  in a "pseudo-R'" in lead V_1 and a pseudo-S wave in the inferior leads (II, III, F).

A **Atrioventricular nodal reentrant tachycardia**

The most common cause (two-thirds of cases) of paroxysmal supraventricular
tachycardia.

Pathophysiology

Requires dual AV nodal pathways (either structurally or functionally distinct).

- One pathway is rapidly conducting and slowly repolarizing (fast path), the other
  is slowly conducting and rapidly repolarizing (slow path) (see Figure 43-1).

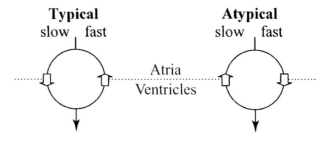

Typical
slow   fast

Atypical
slow   fast

Atria
Ventricles

Usually initiated by an atrial premature contraction, occasionally by a ventricular premature contraction.

May occur in typical or atypical forms.

In typical AVNRT, a premature beat blocks in the fast path and conducts down the slow path. It then conducts to the ventricles and then retrogrades to the atria by reentering the fast pathway distally.

- P-waves may be seen embedded in the terminal QRS forming a "pseudo-S wave" or "pseudo-R" (short R-P).

In atypical AVNRT, a premature beat conducts down the fast path to the ventricles and reenters the slow path distally to travel slowly back to the atria.

- Inverted P-waves seen in the ST segment or T wave (Long R-P).

Differential diagnosis
- Sinus tachycardia (ST)
- AV re-entrant tachycardia (AVRT)
- Atrial flutter (Afl)
- Atrial tachycardia (AT)

P

Admit to a monitored setting

Obtain a cardiology consult

Help determine the diagnosis, if unclear on ECG.

Assist with acute and chronic management.

Attempt to terminate the arrhythmia

If the patient is hemodynamically unstable:
- Perform immediate electrical defibrillation starting at 100 J of energy.

If the patient is hemodynamically stable:
- Perform vagal maneuvers (carotid sinus massage [CSM], Valsalva).

  ◆ CSM should not be performed in patients with carotid bruits or a history of cerebrovascular disease.

- If vagal maneuvers fail, give adenosine (6-mg IV bolus followed by a 12-mg bolus if needed).
- If adenosine fails, give other intravenous AV nodal blocking agent:
  ◆ Diltiazem 10- to 20-mg bolus.
  ◆ Verapamil 5- to 10-mg bolus.
  ◆ Metoprolol 2.5- to 5.0-mg bolus.

Institute chronic medical therapy to prevent recurrences

Patients with only rare episodes can be taught to abort the episode with vagal maneuvers (e.g., Valsalva maneuver, gagging, etc).

For patients with frequent recurrences:
- Chronic administration of AV nodal blocking agents (digoxin, verapamil, diltiazem, or beta-blockers) may be effective.
- Antiarrhythmic agents may be necessary if AV nodal agents fail.
  ◆ Class Ia agents (quinidine, procainamide, disopyramide).
  ◆ Class Ic agents (flecainide, propafenone).
  ◆ Class III agents (amiodarone, sotalol).

Consider definitive therapy with radiofrequency ablation of the reentrant pathway

>90% successful in preventing recurrent AVNRT.

Currently the standard of care for recurrent reentrant arrhythmias.

S **What are the patient's symptoms?**
Common presenting symptoms of ventricular tachycardia (VT) include:
- Lightheadedness
- Syncope
- Sudden cardiac death
- Dizziness
- Palpitations
- Heart failure
- Presyncope
- Chest pain
- Shock

Obtain a medical history
Does the patient have a history of coronary artery disease or myocardial infarction?
Does the patient have a history of other structural heart disease?
- Dilated cardiomyopathy
- Right ventricular dysplasia
- Hypertrophic cardiomyopathy

Does the patient have a family history of arrhythmia or sudden cardiac death?

Is the patient on medications that predispose to ventricular tachyarrhythmias?
Antiarrhythmic agents (quinidine, procainamide, sotalol, digoxin).
Antimicrobial agents (erythromycin, pentamidine, quinolones).
Antipsychotic agents (chlorpromazine, haloperidol, thioridazine).

O **Review vital signs**
Hypotension is common, results from ineffectual cardiac contraction during VT, and requires urgent treatment.

Perform a cardiac examination
Assess for the presence of AV dissociation
- Cannon "a" waves in the jugular venous pressure (JVP) waveform.
  - Cannon "a" waves are prominent pulsations in the JVP resulting from atrial contraction against a closed tricuspid valve.
- Variable intensity of S_1.
Assess for the presence of valvular heart disease or a cardiomyopathy.
- These conditions may predispose to VT.
Assess for evidence of congestive heart failure.
- Congestive heart failure (CHF) may precipitate VT or may be the result of VT.

Obtain a 12-lead ECG
Characteristic findings include:
- Wide complex tachycardia (QRS >120 msec; rate >100 beats per minute).
- AV dissociation (the "P" waves are unrelated to the "QRS" complexes).
- Capture beats ("Dressler beats"): intermittent normal QRS complexes— represent occasional conduction of the atrial impulses to the ventricles.
- Fusion beats: reflect two foci of activation in the heart and confirm VT.

Request a chemistry panel
Renal dysfunction and electrolyte abnormalities (especially potassium and magnesium) can predispose to VT.

Ventricular tachycardia
Defined as ≥3 consecutive ventricular beats at a rate of >100/min.
If the rhythm terminates spontaneously in <30 seconds it is termed nonsustained VT (NSVT). NSVT is often asymptomatic.
Monomorphic VT has a monotonous QRS morphology and usually reflects a reentrant circuit through abnormal myocardium (e.g., prior myocardial infarction [MI]).
Polymorphic VT refers to a varying QRS morphology during the tachycardia.
 • Suggests either acute ischemia, drug toxicity, or long QT syndrome.

Differential diagnosis
Supraventricular tachycardia with aberrancy
AV re-entrant tachycardia (i.e., a bypass tract)
Pacemaker mediated tachycardia

 Follow ACLS protocols for patients with sustained VT
If the patient is hypotensive or becomes pulseless:
 • Immediately defibrillate using between 100 and 300 J of energy.
 • Begin CPR if required, and stabilize the airway.
If the patient is hemodynamically stable, consider chemical cardioversion:
 • Amiodarone 150 mg IV bolus over 5 minutes, then 1 mg/min for 6 hours, then 0.5 mg/min for 18 hours.
 • Lidocaine 1 mg/kg IV bolus, then 1 to 4 mg/min infusion.

Admit the patient to the coronary care unit when stabilized

Obtain cardiology consultation

Identify and treat the etiology of the VT
Correct electrolyte abnormalities: Keep potassium >4 and magnesium >2.
Treat ischemia with aspirin, nitrates, beta-blockers, and heparin.
Treat CHF with diuretics, angiotensin-converting enzyme inhibitors, and beta-blockers.
Stop medications that may prolong the QT interval.

Check serial cardiac enzymes to exclude acute MI
Start β-blocker therapy (e.g., metoprolol 25 mg bid) unless contraindicated.

Obtain an echocardiogram
The long-term management of VT depends in part on the LV function.
Assess overall LV ejection fraction.
Assess for evidence of prior MI or valvular dysfunction.

Consider stress testing in patients with suspected coronary artery disease (CAD) and normal left ventricular ejection fraction (LVEF)

Consider cardiac catheterization in patients with suspected CAD and LVEF <50% or with an abnormal stress test
Coronary revascularization should be performed if possible.

Consider placement of an implantable cardioverter defibrillator in patients with:
Sudden cardiac death and an LVEF <35%.
Prior MI and an LVEF <30%.
Nonischemic cardiomyopathy with LVEF <30% and recurrent VT/NSVT.

S **Does the patient have symptoms related to high blood pressure (BP)?**
Most patients with hypertension (HTN) are asymptomatic.
Potential symptoms include:
- Headache
- Visual changes
- Chest pain
- Dyspnea
- Palpitations
- Neurological symptoms

Are there any dietary or social habits contributing to hypertension?
- High sodium intake
- Substance abuse (alcohol, tobacco, cocaine)
- Medications (oral contraceptives, decongestants, steroids)

Does the patient have characteristics to suggest secondary causes of hypertension?
Age of onset <20 years or >50 years.
Refractory hypertension despite multiple medications.
Paroxysms of elevated BP precipitating heart failure.

Enquire about the following comorbidities that may affect management
- Diabetes
- Chronic obstructive pulmonary disease
- Pregnancy
- Coronary artery disease (CAD)
- Renal disease
- Congestive heart failure (CHF)
- Prostatic hypertrophy

O **Check the patient's blood pressure**
BP should be obtained in both arms with the patient sitting and at rest.
Inflate cuff until the radial pulse is not palpable, then deflate 2 to 3 mm Hg/sec.
- The first Korotkoff sound is the systolic BP.
- The fifth (last) Korotkoff sound is the diastolic BP.
Make sure that the BP cuff is the correct size.
- An undersized cuff will overestimate BP.

Perform a funduscopic examination to evaluate for hypertensive retinopathy
- Grade I: arterial narrowing
- Grade III: hemorrhages and exudates
- Grade II: arteriovenous nicking
- Grade IV: papilledema

Examine the heart
A laterally displaced point of maximal impulse may be indicative of hypertensive cardiomyopathy.
- The left ventricle tends to hypertrophy initially and eventually dilates.
A loud S_2 reflects rapid closure of the AV due to elevated BP.
An S_4 reflects atrial contraction into a poorly compliant left ventricle.
Mitral or aortic regurgitant murmurs are common with severe HTN.

Listen for vascular bruits
Hypertension is a major risk factor for developing vascular disease.

Perform a neurologic assessment
Hypertension can cause hemorrhagic or ischemic strokes.

Look for signs of secondary hypertension (see SOAP 46)

Perform electrocardiography
Look for left ventricular hypertrophy, a "strain pattern," or evidence of ischemia/infarction.

Perform urine analysis and serum tests of renal function
Microalbuminuria, elevated blood urea nitrogen, or creatinine reflects renal damage.

A **Essential hypertension**
Hypertension that occurs in the absence of an identifiable cause. Classified according to the 7th Joint National Commission on Hypertension (JNC VII) (Table 45-1):

Table 45-1	Hypertension Classification	
Blood Pressure Classification	Systolic Blood Pressure (mm Hg)	Diastolic Blood Pressure (mm Hg)
Normal	<120	And <80
Prehypertension	120–139	Or 80–89
Stage I hypertension	140–159	Or 90–99
Stage II hypertension	>160	Or >100

P

Obtain serial blood pressure measurements
Elevated BP must be documented on 2 or more measurements during 2 or more evaluations before diagnosing a patient with HTN.

Assess for end-organ damage
- Retinopathy   - Left ventricular hypertrophy   - CHF
- CAD   - Vascular disease   - Renal insufficiency

Encourage lifestyle modification in all patients
- Weight loss   - <2 g sodium intake per day
- Decrease alcohol intake   - Aerobic exercise
- Smoking cessation   - Avoid medications that may elevate BP

Institute pharmacologic therapy depending on severity of HTN
Patients with stage I HTN with no cardiac risk factors or end organ damage:
- Consider a 6-month trial of lifestyle modification.
- Start anti-HTN medication if BP remains elevated after this period.

Patients with stage I HTN with cardiac risk factors (especially diabetes) or end organ damage, and patients with stage II HTN:
- Start thiazide diuretic unless compelling indication for other therapy.   ± ARB
- Two-drug therapy may be required as initial therapy for stage II HTN.

Evaluate for compelling indications for specific anti-hypertensive therapy
Diabetes: angiotensin-converting enzyme inhibitor (ACEI)/angiotensin receptor blocker.
CAD: beta-blocker, ACEI.
Systolic heart failure: beta-blocker, ACEI.
Diastolic heart failure: beta-blocker, ACEI, calcium channel blocker.
Renal disease: diuretic, ACEI (if creatinine <3).
Pregnancy: hydralazine, methyldopa.
Chronic obstructive pulmonary disease: ACEI (avoid beta-blocker).
Prostatic hypertrophy: alpha-blocker.

Follow BP every 1–2 weeks until goal BP achieved

Start medications at lower doses and up-titrate every 1 to 2 weeks until goal achieved
Goal BP: <140/90 mm Hg for patients with uncomplicated HTN.
             <130/80 mm Hg for patients with diabetes mellitus, CAD, chronic renal disease.
If BP not at goal after maximization of initial agent, add a second agent of a different class.

Evaluate for secondary causes of HTN in appropriate patients. (See SOAP 46.)

S **Does the patient have clinical features suggestive of a secondary cause of hypertension (HTN)?**

Severe HTN (systolic BP >180 mm Hg; diastolic BP >110 mm Hg).

HTN resistant to treatment despite 4 or more antihypertensive agents.

Age at onset of HTN <20 years or >50 years.

Abrupt onset of severe HTN, especially with renal dysfunction.

Rapid worsening of BP after a period of good control.

Progressive renal dysfunction after institution of an ACE inhibitor.

Does the patient have symptoms attributable to HTN?

Patients with secondary HTN are frequently symptomatic.

Usual symptoms are similar to those of essential HTN. (See SOAP 45.)

Symptoms specifically suggestive of a secondary cause of HTN include:

- Flushing
- Pruritus
- Anxiety
- Polyuria
- Weight loss
- Hyperhidrosis
- Diarrhea
- Palpitations

♦ These symptoms are often caused by excessive neurohormonal secretion or renal dysfunction.

Does the patient have a family history of inheritable causes of secondary HTN?

Polycystic kidney disease.

Graves disease.

Pheochromocytoma (may occur as part of the Multiple Endocrine Neoplasia (MEN) syndrome, type II; or von Hippel-Lindau syndrome).

Does the patient take medications or other substances that may exacerbate HTN?

- Decongestants
- Alcohol
- Steroids
- Cocaine
- Oral contraceptives
- Amphetamines

Does the patient use an excessive amount of sodium in their diet?

O **Assess serial blood pressure values**

Consider 24-hour BP monitoring.

- Extreme paroxysms of HTN are suspicious for a secondary cause.

Check BP in both arms and in the lower extremities

- Systolic BP higher in the right arm than in the left arm, or higher in the arms than in the legs suggests aortic coarctation.

Inspect for overt signs of secondary HTN

Pale, sallow skin may be indicative of renal parenchymal disease.

Striae, a buffalo hump, or a moon face suggest Cushing's syndrome.

Pallor, tremor, and sweating suggest pheochromocytoma.

Goiter, proptosis, or myxedema indicate thyroid dysfunction.

Hirsutism and obesity are often present with polycystic kidney disease.

Perform a thorough cardiovascular examination

A left precordial or interscapular systolic murmur suggests aortic coarctation.

A pericardial friction rub may be present in patients with renal disease.

Abdominal bruits or evidence of peripheral vascular disease (e.g., femoral or carotid bruits, diminished pedal pulses) suggests renovascular disease.

Perform an abdominal examination

Palpable kidneys are often appreciated in polycystic kidney disease.

Secondary hypertension
Refers to HTN resulting from an identifiable cause. Accounts for only 5% to 10% of HTN.

Etiologies
Endocrine: Conn's syndrome, Cushing's syndrome, pheochromocytoma, acromegaly, hyperparathyroidism, hyper- or hypothyroidism.
Renal: Renal artery stenosis, fibromuscular dysplasia, parenchymal disease (polycystic kidney disease, polyarteritis nodosa, glomerulonephritis, etc).
Vascular: Aortic coarctation, vasculitis.
Miscellaneous: Obstructive sleep apnea, high salt diet, oral contraceptive pills, monoamine oxidase inhibitors, corticosteroids, alcohol, substance abuse.

Obtain routine laboratory tests
Combination of hypokalemia, mild hypernatremia, and alkalosis suggests hyperaldosteronism.
Elevated BUN and creatinine suggests renal vascular or parenchymal disease.

Perform specific laboratory tests appropriate to the history and physical findings
Thyroid profile to exclude thyroid disease.
Cortisol stimulation test for Cushing's disease.
Plasma renin and aldosterone levels for hyperaldosteronism.
24-hour urinary vanillylmandelic acid and metanephrine levels to identify pheochromocytoma; serum levels of metanephrines may be preferred.
24-hour urinary protein and creatinine levels, and creatinine clearance to assess renal parenchymal disease.

Consider further tests or imaging modalities based on the specific cause suspected
Aortic coarctation: may be seen on echocardiogram; computed tomography (CT) or magnetic resonance imaging (MRI) of the chest are the tests of choice.
Pheochromocytoma: abdominal CT scan or I-MIBG (radionucleotide) scan.
Renovascular disease: magnetic resonance angiography or renal angiogram.
Hyperaldosteronism: abdominal CT scan to evaluate for adrenal adenoma.
Cushing's disease: head CT or MRI to exclude pituitary adenoma.

Institute therapy directed at the specific secondary cause of HTN present
Renovascular disease: percutaneous or surgical renal artery revascularization.
Hyperaldosteronism: resection of adrenal adenomas; spironolactone should be used in patients with bilateral adrenal hyperplasia.
Cushing's syndrome: resection of causative pituitary or adrenal tumor.
Pheochromocytoma: medical treatment with phenoxybenzamine until surgical resection of the tumor can be performed.
Aortic coarctation: surgical or percutaneous correction of the coarctation.
Thyroid replacement for hypothyroidism.
Thyroid resection or ablation (with radioactivity) for hyperthyroidism.

Counsel all patients with regard to necessary dietary and lifestyle changes
- Sodium restriction   - Weight loss   - Increased physical activity
- Avoidance of oral contraceptive agents, alcohol, and recreational drugs

S **How high is the patient's blood pressure?**
A BP of >230/130 mm Hg is considered a hypertensive crisis.

Does patient have symptoms of acute end organ damage?
Chest pain from cardiac ischemia or aortic dissection.
Shortness of breath from congestive heart failure or cardiac ischemia.
Visual changes (blurry vision, scotomata) from retinal involvement.
Neurologic symptoms (headache, confusion, slurred speech, weakness, vision loss)
from cerebral ischemia, intracranial hemorrhage, or hypertensive encephalopathy.
Hematuria, frothy urine, or oliguria from glomerular disease.

Does the patient have a history of hypertension?
Lack of preceding hypertension should prompt an evaluation for a secondary
cause.
Patients with chronic hypertension may better tolerate severe hypertension.

Is the patient compliant with hypertensive therapy and dietary restrictions?
Rebound hypertension (HTN) may occur after acute discontinuation of clonidine or
beta-blockers.
Severe hypertension can occur after a sodium rich meal.

Take a thorough medication and illicit drug history
Alcohol, cocaine, decongestants, "herbal" stimulants, and steroids can cause severe
HTN.

 Review the vital signs
Check manual blood pressure in both arms. Ensure appropriate cuff size is used.
● Discrepant blood pressure in the arms is concerning for aortic dissection or
previously undiagnosed aortic coarctation.
A widened pulse pressure may suggest aortic insufficiency complicating a
dissection.
Bradycardia in the setting of severe hypertension suggests increased intracranial
pressure (Cushing's reflex).

Perform a physical examination
Funduscopic examination: Look for hemorrhages, exudates, and papilledema.
Cardiac examination: Listen for S_3, S_4 or the diastolic murmur of aortic
insufficiency.
Pulmonary examination: Listen for signs of heart failure.
Vascular examination.
● Listen for bruits in the carotid, vertebral, subclavian and femoral arteries.
● Feel for enlargement of the abdominal aorta and listen for abdominal bruits.
Neurologic examination: Assess mental status and look for focal neurological
deficits.

Obtain an electrocardiogram
Review for evidence of ventricular hypertrophy and for acute ischemia.

Review the chest radiograph for evidence of
A widened mediastinum suggesting aortic dissection.
Pulmonary edema.

Review laboratory tests to evaluate for evidence of end organ damage
Blood urea nitrogen and creatinine.
Complete blood cell count (?hemolysis resulting from hypertensive vasculitis).
Cardiac enzymes in patients with suspicious symptoms.
Urinalysis to assess for hematuria and proteinuria.

Obtain head CT or MRI if hemorrhagic or ischemic stoke is suspected

Obtain chest CT, chest MRI, or transesophageal echocardiograph if aortic dissection is suspected

Hypertensive emergency

Defined as markedly elevated BP with evidence of acute end-organ damage (cardiovascular, renal, neurological, or ophthalmologic). Immediate BP lowering is required, usually with parenteral medications.

Markedly elevated blood pressure without evidence of end-organ damage is referred to as hypertensive urgency.

Admit the patient to the intensive care unit

Consider use of an intraarterial catheter for continuous blood pressure monitoring.

Administer parenteral antihypertensive agents to acutely lower the BP

Goal of treatment should be a 25% reduction in mean arterial pressure (MAP) within the first 30 to 60 minutes (MAP = 2/3 × diastolic pressure + 1/3 × systolic pressure).
- More rapid reductions in MAP may result in cerebral hypoperfusion.
- Gradually return blood pressure toward normal over several days.

Choose a specific parenteral agent depending on the clinical setting

Labetalol: 15- to 40-mg bolus followed by an infusion at 0.5 to 2 mg/minute.
- A combined alpha- and beta-adrenergic antagonist: onset within 5 to 10 minutes.
- Drug of choice in aortic dissection and most hypertensive emergencies.
- Avoid in acute congestive heart failure, atrioventricular block, moderate-to-severe asthma.

Sodium nitroprusside: 0.25 to 0.5 μg/kg/min and titrate to 10 μg/kg/min.
- Arterial and venous vasodilator- onset within seconds; offset within minutes.
- Dose limited by accumulation of cyanide metabolites after 24–48 hours.
- Avoid in aortic dissection unless co-administered with beta-blockers.
- May increase intracranial pressure.

Nitroglycerin: 5 μg/min and titrate up to 300 μg/min to achieve goal BP.
- Venous > arterial vasodilator: onset and offset similar to nitroprusside.
- Drug of choice in ischemic heart disease and acute CHF.

Nicardipine: 5 to 15 mg/hr.
- Parenteral dihydropyridine calcium channel blocker.
- Good choice when hypertensive emergency is complicated by subarachnoid hemorrhage (prevents cerebral vasospasm).

Hydralazine: 20 mg IV—direct-acting arterial vasodilator.
- Primarily indicated for use in pregnancy/pre-eclampsia.
- Avoid in coronary disease or aortic dissection without concurrent beta-blocker.

Fenoldopam: start 1 μg/kg/min and titrate every 15 minutes as needed.
- Peripheral dopamine-1 receptor agonist—maintains or increases renal perfusion.
- Safe for all hypertensive emergencies.
- Contraindicated in patients with glaucoma.

Phentolamine: 5- to 10-mg IV bolus.
- Alpha-adrenergic antagonist.
- Indicated in catecholamine excess (pheochromocytoma or tyramine ingestion in a patient on an MAO inhibitor).

Esmolol: parenteral beta-blocker with very short half-life; allows rapid titration.

Initiate oral therapy once BP stabilized

Evaluate for secondary causes of hypertension (see SOAP 46)

S **What are the patient's current symptoms?**

Aortic dissection classically presents with sharp, tearing pain that radiates to the back.
May also present with syncope, paralysis, heart failure, abdominal pain, or limb pain.
- These symptoms reflect critical organ ischemia as a result of impaired flow in
  the vascular branches of the aorta.
10% of cases may be asymptomatic.

Does the patient have risk factors for aortic dissection?

- HTN
- Bicuspid aortic valve
- Pregnancy
- Cocaine abuse
- Iatrogenic causes (e.g., recent
  cardiac catheterization or coronary bypass surgery)
- Atherosclerosis
- Collagen vascular disorders (e.g., Marfan's
  syndrome)
- Tertiary syphilis
- Chest trauma (e.g., motor vehicle accident)

Does the patient have a history of aortic disease?

Patients with aortic aneurysms or prior aortic dissection are at increased risk of subsequent dissection.

Obtain a list of medications and assess medication compliance

Decongestants, monoamine oxidase inhibitors, oral contraceptives, herbal supple-
ments, cocaine, and alcohol can all cause severe HTN with resultant dissection.
Medication noncompliance, and sudden cessation of clonidine and beta-blockers
may lead to rebound hypertension and predispose to aortic dissection.

Perform a general review of symptoms

May identify symptoms of organ dysfunction related to the aortic dissection.
May suggest alternate diagnoses (e.g., esophageal spasm, gastroesophageal reflux
disease, peptic ulcer disease, pericarditis).

 Check pulse and blood pressure in all extremities

Patients with descending aortic dissections are often hypertensive while patients with
ascending dissections are frequently hypotensive (due to acute AI or tamponade).
Hypertension and tachycardia may hasten propagation of the dissection and warrant
immediate treatment.
Asymmetric pressure or absent pulses are classic signs of aortic dissection.

Perform a physical examination paying special attention to

Presence of aortic insufficiency.
- Suggests that the dissection involves the ascending aorta and aortic valve.
Signs of cardiac tamponade (increased jugular venous pressure, pulsus paradox).
(See SOAP 20.)
- Suggests rupture of the aorta into the pericardial space.
Carotid bruits: may indicate vascular compromise and increased risk of stroke.
Altered mental status and motor or sensory deficits.
Signs of limb ischemia.

Obtain a chest radiograph

Characteristic abnormalities include a widened mediastinum, tracheal deviation,
pleural effusion, diffuse enlargement of the descending thoracic aorta.

Perform electrocardiography

Exclude myocardial ischemia or infarction as the cause of chest pain.
- Right coronary artery involvement (inferior ST elevation) common with
  ascending dissections.

A
Aortic dissection
Results from a tear in the aortic intima that allows blood to enter the subintimal space, separating the intima from the media and creating an intimal flap. Propagation of the dissection impairs blood flow down branch vessels. Pathophysiology appears to be cystic medial necrosis.

Variants of aortic dissection
Class I: classic dissection with dual lumen and intimal flap.
Class II: intramural hematoma without an intimal flap.
Class III: intimal tear without hematoma (limited dissection).
Class IV: penetrating aortic ulcer.
Class V: iatrogenic/traumatic dissection.

Classification of aortic dissection
Stanford type A: Dissection involving the ascending aorta regardless of site of tear.
Stanford type B: Dissection involving the descending aorta only.

Differential diagnosis
- Myocardial ischemia/infarction   - Pulmonary embolism   - Acute pericarditis
- Peptic ulcer disease   - Esophageal spasm   - Musculoskeletal pain

P
Confirm the diagnosis with transesophageal echocardiography (TEE), contrast-enhanced computed tomography (CT), or magnetic resonance imaging (MRI)
All are >90% sensitive and specific for the diagnosis.
Choice of test depends on availability and institutional expertise.
- MRI allows visualization of the entire aorta and its branches and is least invasive. Requires the most time—difficult to use in the acute setting.
- Spiral CT is rapid but requires IV contrast.
- TEE is invasive, but can be performed at the bedside. This is the study of choice in a hemodynamically unstable patient.

Obtain emergent thoracic surgical consult when aortic dissection is diagnosed

Proceed to emergent surgery for type A dissections
Higher complication risk including stroke, aortic insufficiency, and tamponade.
Mortality rate approaches 1% per hour during the first 48 hours.
- Mortality is significantly reduced by surgical therapy.
Requires repair of the ascending aorta and repair/replacement of the AV if involved.
Initiate beta-blocker therapy while awaiting surgery, unless hypotension is present.

Institute medical therapy for type B dissections
Lower risk of complications and mortality than type A dissection.
Lower mortality with medical management than with surgical management.
Admit to ICU.
Control hypertension with intravenous medications.
- Beta-blockers should be used routinely (e.g., labetalol, metoprolol).
  ◆ Reduce dP/dT and heart rate and limit propagation of the dissection.
- Add vasodilators as needed (e.g., nitroprusside, enalaprilat).
Aim for goal BP ~120/80 mm Hg.
Surgical repair may be required for limb ischemia or dissection propagation.

Control chest pain with analgesia and avoid all anticoagulants

Repeat diagnostic study if suspect propagation of dissection or new organ/limb ischemia

S **Does the patient have claudication?**
Claudication (ischemic muscle pain) is the most common symptom of peripheral
arterial disease (PAD).

What muscles are affected?
The location of symptoms depends on the effected vascular supply:
- Femoral or popliteal artery disease → thigh/calf claudication.
- Tibial or peroneal artery disease → foot claudication.
- Aorto-iliac artery disease → buttock, hip, and/or thigh claudication.
- Subclavian artery disease → arm claudication.

Are there aggravating or alleviating factors?
Symptoms are usually precipitated by exertion and relieved with rest.
With more advanced disease, symptoms may occur at rest or during sleep.
Rest pain may be relieved by hanging the feet over the edge of the bed.

Does the patient have risk factors for vascular disease?
Diabetes mellitus, hypertension, dyslipidemia, cigarette smoking.
Age (male >45 years, female >55 years), family history of premature coronary artery
disease.
Other risk factors include homocysteinemia, obesity, inactivity.

Does the patient have symptoms or a history of other vascular disease?
Coronary artery disease (angina, myocardial infarction).
- 50% of patients with PAD have significant coronary artery disease.
Cerebrovascular disease (stroke, transient ischemic attack).

O **Check vital signs**
Poorly controlled BP in patients with PAD may indicate renal artery stenosis.
Check BP in both arms to exclude subclavian stenosis.

Perform a thorough vascular examination
Examine carotid, radial, abdominal aortic, femoral, popliteal, and pedal pulses.
Pulses will be decreased or absent distal to the vascular obstruction.
Vascular bruits may be heard over the diseased arteries.

Look for cutaneous signs of vascular disease
Hair loss, smooth and shiny skin, thickened nails.

Look for signs of limb ischemia
Chronic limb ischemia may result in pallor, cyanosis, and dependent rubor of the
limb.
Ulcers or gangrene may be noted in severe disease.
Acute limb ischemia usually presents with pain, pallor, pulselessness, paresthesias,
paralysis, and poikilothermia.

Obtain an electrocardiogram
Look for evidence of coronary artery disease.

 Peripheral artery disease
Atherosclerotic disease of the peripheral arteries results in vascular narrowing,
limitation of distal blood flow, and reduction in oxygen delivery to the affected
limb, thereby producing ischemic symptoms.

Differential diagnosis
Other causes of true claudication (vasculitis, thromboangiitis obliterans, vasospasm;
or acute arterial obstruction due to aortic dissection, embolus, or trauma).
Pseudoclaudication: results from lumbar spinal stenosis.

- Produces exertional pain similar to arterial claudication.
- Unlike true claudication, the relief of pseudoclaudication requires not only the cessation of activity, but also a change in position (i.e., sitting).
- Nonischemic pain, musculoskeletal pain.

Prognosis
5-year mortality of patients with claudication: 30%.
5-year risk of amputation: 5% overall, 20% in diabetics, 50% in active smokers.

P

Obtain a study to quantify the severity of PAD
Ankle brachial index (ABI): Segmental BPs in the leg are compared to brachial pressure. The systolic pressure in the leg is usually equal or slightly greater than the arm (ABI >1.0). An ABI <1.0 indicates PAD and the location of the fall in BP suggests the region of stenosis.
- ABI 0.80 to 1.0: mild disease.
- ABI 0.5 to 0.80: moderate disease.
- ABI <0.50: severe disease.

Pulse volume recordings (PVR): Pulsatile volume changes in the legs are translated into a pressure curve. The amplitude of the pulse wave falls in the presence of PAD.
Doppler flow velocity—similar to PVR; flow velocity falls with progressive PAD.
Contrast angiography or magnetic resonance angiography (MRA)—used to assess the location and severity of PVD, usually in preparation for revascularization.

Institute aggressive risk factor modification in all patients with PAD
Smoking cessation, lipid lowering therapy, control of hypertension and diabetes.
Exercise, specifically walking, has been shown to improve exercise capacity.

Institute medical therapy for PAD
Antiplatelet therapy.
- Aspirin (81 to 325 mg qd) is indicated in all patients with PAD.
- Use clopidogrel (75 mg qd) in aspirin-allergic patients.

Cilostazol (a phosphodiesterase inhibitor; 100 mg bid).
- Antiplatelet and vasodilator effects.
- The most effective agent for increasing walk time in patients with PAD.

Lipid lowering therapy (statins).
- Decreases claudication, reduces cerebrovascular events in patients with PAD.

Pentoxifylline decreases blood viscosity. Minimal effect on symptoms.

Consider revascularization
For patients with rest pain, ischemic ulcers, gangrene, or unacceptable symptoms.
Can be performed either surgically or percutaneously.
- Percutaneous revascularization with stent placement is useful for iliac arteries but less effective for more distal disease.
- Surgical revascularization is effective for aortic, iliac, and femoral disease but less efficacious for more distal disease.

Consider evaluation for carotid artery disease as well as cardiac stress testing given the high prevalence of vascular disease in other sites

Does the patient have a history of hypertension?
The most common finding of aortic coarctation is HTN, often beginning in childhood.

Does the patient have symptoms attributable to aortic coarctation?
Most patients with coarctation are asymptomatic—diagnosis is made on examination.
When present, symptoms usually result from severe hypertension.
- Headache
- Epistaxis
- Chest pain
- Heart failure
- Stroke
- Lower extremity claudication

Neonates with coarctation may present in severe heart failure and/or shock when the ductus arteriosus and foramen ovale begin to close.

Does the patient have a history of a murmur in childhood?
Coarctation is frequently associated with other congenital cardiac abnormalities.
- Bicuspid aortic valve (~50% co-incidence).
- Ventricular septal defect.
- Patent ductus arteriosus.
- Aortic and mitral stenosis.

Does the patient have other conditions associated with coarctation?
Gonadal dysgenesis (Turner's syndrome).
Aneurysms of the Circle of Willis.

O Perform a directed review of systems
Search for symptoms of hypertension or vascular insufficiency.

Check the patient's blood pressure and pulse in all four extremities
Isolated upper extremity hypertension is the classic finding of aortic coarctation.
In coarctation of the aortic arch hypertension may be limited to the right arm only.
The femoral pulse is usually delayed when compared to the radial or carotid pulse.

Perform a thorough cardiac examination looking for the following features
Mid-systolic murmur at the left sternal border and left interscapular area due to flow across the coarctation.
Continuous murmur over the upper chest and posterior ribs due to flow through a patent ductus arteriosus and large collateral vessels.
An ejection systolic click and systolic ejection murmur of a bicuspid aortic valve.
Palpable and sustained LV impulse due to hypertension, and palpable pulsations in the intercostal spaces from large collateral arteries to the lower body.

Obtain an electrocardiogram
Usually suggests left ventricular hypertrophy from longstanding hypertension.

Obtain a chest radiograph
Classic findings include:
- Notching of the inferior aspects of ribs 3 to 8 due to collateral vessel formation.
- Dilation of the aorta proximal and distal to the site of coarctation producing the "reverse E" or "3" sign.

Aortic coarctation

Pathophysiology
Usually a congenital, discrete narrowing at the proximal thoracic aorta just distal to the origin of the left subclavian artery, at the site of the ligamentum arteriosum. Less commonly it may be proximal to the left (and rarely the right) subclavian artery. The coarctation results in upper extremity hypertension that is fueled by neurohormonal mediators (renin-angiotensin) released as a result of renal artery hypoperfusion.

Epidemiology
Congenital aortic coarctation is 2–5 times more common in males than in females.

Differential diagnosis
Acquired coarctation associated with Takayasu's arteritis or severe atherosclerosis.

Prognosis
Congestive heart failure occurs in two thirds of patients older than the age of 40 who have an uncorrected coarctation.
Other complications include aortic dissection, endocarditis, cerebral hemorrhage.
90% of patients with an uncorrected coarctation die by the age of 60 years.

P

Obtain a definitive imaging study
Echocardiogram:
- Can confirm the diagnosis and estimate the pressure gradient across the coarctation.
- Can assess for associated cardiac and vascular abnormalities.

Aortography, magnetic resonance angiography, and computed tomography angiography:
- Can visualize the exact location and length on the involved aortic segment.
- May visualize collateral vessels.

Treat infants with coarctation-related congestive heart failure with aggressive medical management
Intravenous infusion of prostaglandin E_1 to keep the ductus arteriosus patent.
Pressors/inotropic agents as needed to support the BP.
Diuretics to treat pulmonary edema.
Surgery or balloon angioplasty can be performed after stabilization.

Consider aortic repair in children and adults if the pressure gradient across the coarctation is >30 mm Hg
Surgery is the preferred approach.
- Coarctation resection and reanastomosis of the aorta is the usual approach.
- Left subclavian to distal aortic bypass is an alternative technique.

Percutaneous balloon dilation and stenting is an alternative to surgery.

Perform serial examinations of patients after coarctation repair
Recurrent coarctation occurs more commonly after balloon dilation than with surgery.
- Consider repeat imaging study in patients with increasing murmur intensity or recurrent HTN.

Monitor blood pressure and treat HTN aggressively.
- Resolution of HTN is influenced by the patient's age at the time of repair.
- Residual hypertension is rare when repair is performed in early childhood (90% are normotensive 5 years after surgery).
- If repair is after age 40, approximately 50% of patients remain hypertensive.
- Normotensive patients often have exaggerated HTN during exercise.

Prescribe antibiotic prophylaxis to prevent endocarditis in all patients with coarctation

S **Does the patient have any symptoms related to carotid artery disease?**

Carefully ask about any prior neurologic symptoms.
- Patients with prior transient ischemic attack (TIA) (see SOAP 52) or stroke (see SOAP 53) are treated much differently than patients with asymptomatic carotid disease.

Common symptoms of carotid disease include:
- Slurred speech
- Visual blurring
- Transient visual loss
- Facial droop
- Arm, hand, or leg weakness

Does the patient have symptoms of coronary or peripheral arterial disease?
Carotid disease is often a marker of diffuse vascular disease.

Does the patient have risk factors for atherosclerotic vascular disease?
- Diabetes mellitus
- Hypertension
- Dyslipidemia
- Cigarette smoking
- Obesity
- Hyperhomocystinemia
- Age (male >45 years; female >55 years)
- Family history of premature vascular disease (male <55 years; female <60 years)

O **Review vital signs**
Hypertension is often present.

Perform a directed physical examination focusing on the following
Funduscopic examination:
- Hypertensive retinopathy
- Hollenhorst plaques (cholesterol emboli)

Vascular examination:
- Listen for bruits in the carotid, vertebral, subclavian, and femoral arteries.
  - A bruit is the sound made by turbulent flow through a stenosed artery.
- Feel for enlargement of the abdominal aorta and listen for abdominal bruits.

Cardiac examination:
- Listen for an aortic valve murmur, which may radiate to the carotids and mimic a carotid bruit.

Extremity examination:
- Look for evidence of peripheral vascular disease, such as diminished distal pulses, cool extremities, hair loss, and trophic skin and nail changes.

Neurologic examination:
- Mental status
- Speech
- Cranial nerves
- Strength
- Sensory exam
- Reflexes
- Gait

  - Neurologic deficits may indicate prior stroke (i.e., not asymptomatic).

Review the patient's electrocardiogram
Look for evidence of concomitant coronary artery disease (ischemia or infarction).

Obtain a fasting lipid panel

A **Asymptomatic carotid bruit**
Only ~35% of patients with a carotid bruit have a significant carotid stenosis.
Only 50% of patients with significant carotid stenosis have a carotid bruit.
A carotid bruit is a much stronger marker of diffuse vascular disease than a
predictor of subsequent neurologic event.

Differential diagnosis
- Vertebral artery stenosis
- Thyroid bruit (usually in setting of thyrotoxicosis)
- Radiated murmur from aortic stenosis
- Venous hum of pregnancy

P **Consider obtaining an imaging study to confirm the presence of a carotid stenosis and assess its severity**
Carotid artery duplex ultrasound.
Magnetic resonance angiography (MRA).
- Both can confirm the presence of carotid stenosis and quantify its severity.
- Have similar sensitivity (~85%) and specificity (~90%) for identifying carotid a stenosis of >70%.
Contrast angiography.
- Invasive, but is the gold standard for identifying carotid stenoses.
- Usually reserved for patients who are undergoing endarterectomy.
Unclear if these tests change therapy or long-term outcome in asymptomatic patients.

Aggressively manage risk factors
Smoking cessation: reduces the risk of subsequent stroke.
Blood pressure control: reduces the risk of subsequent stroke.
Glycemic control: indicated but of unproven benefit for stroke reduction.
Lipid lowering therapy: ~25% reduction in subsequent stroke.

Consider treatment with aspirin
No clear reduction in stroke risk in asymptomatic patients, but may be indicated for primary prevention of myocardial infarction.
Strongly consider use in patients with multiple risk factors and low bleeding risk.

Consider referring to a vascular surgeon
Can assist with weighing risks and benefits of surgical therapy in a given patient.

Consider carotid endarterectomy
Of proven benefit in patients with *symptomatic* carotid stenosis of >70%.
May be of benefit in asymptomatic patients with >60% carotid stenosis, but only if performed by an experienced surgeon.
- Acceptable rate of perioperative complication: <3%.
Percutaneous endovascular carotid stenting has not been studied in patients with asymptomatic carotid stenosis.

S

What are the patient's symptoms?
Symptoms of a transient ischemic attack (TIA) usually develop suddenly and may include:
- Unilateral leg, arm, and/or facial weakness or heaviness
- Unilateral paresthesias, either alone or in combination with a motor deficit.
- Visual abnormalities including transient monocular blindness (Amaurosis fugax), diplopia, or blurring of vision.
- Vertigo or ataxia.
- Dysarthria or dysphagia.
- Aphasia and/or agnosia.

How long have the symptoms lasted?
By definition, TIAs last <24 hours and resolve completely without residual deficit.

Has the patient had similar symptoms in the past?
Recurrent TIAs that produce the same neurologic deficit suggest focal arterial disease. Recurrent TIAs with varying deficits suggest either embolic disease from the heart, aorta, or great vessels; or diffuse disease of the cranial arteries.

Does the patient have risk factors for atherosclerotic vascular disease?
- Diabetes mellitus
- Tobacco use
- Dyslipidemia
- Hypertension
- Age (male >45 years; female >55 years)
- Family history of premature coronary artery disease or vascular disease (male <55 years; female <60 years)

Does the patient have conditions associated with emboli from the heart or great vessels?
- Dilated cardiomyopathy
- Known carotid artery disease
- Intracardiac shunts (patent foramen ovale, atrial septal defect, ventricular septal defect)
- Atrial fibrillation
- Endocarditis

Does the patient have a hyperviscosity or hypercoagulable syndrome?
- Sickle cell disease
- Monoclonal gammopathies
- Protein C or S deficiency
- Lupus anticoagulant/Antiphospholipid antibody
- Polycythemia or thrombocytosis
- Antithrombin III deficiency
- Hyperhomocystinemia

O

Perform a physical examination
Vital signs: Irregular pulse may indicate atrial fibrillation.
Funduscopic examination: May reveal evidence of hypertensive retinopathy or "Hollenhorst" plaques (bright yellow cholesterol emboli).
Cardiac examination: An irregularly irregular rhythm suggests atrial fibrillation; regurgitant murmurs may suggest endocarditis; an S_3 may suggest a cardiomyopathy.
Vascular examination: Listen carefully for carotid bruits.
Extremity examination: Look for evidence of peripheral embolization (digital ischemia) or manifestations of endocarditis (splinter hemorrhages, petechiae).
Neurologic examination: Assess mental status, speech, cranial nerves, strength, gait, reflexes, sensory examination, position and vibration sense.

- Serial neurologic examinations are essential to assess the presence and time course of resolution of symptoms.

Transient ischemic attack
The sudden onset of focal neurological symptoms and/or signs that lasts less than 24 hours. Pathophysiology relates to a transient decrease in regional cerebral blood supply resulting from atherosclerosis of the cerebral circulation, embolization from the heart or extracranial vessels, or hypertensive cerebrovascular disease.

Differential diagnosis
Subarachnoid or intracranial hemorrhage may mimic TIA, although symptoms are usually less transient and excluded by computed tomography scan.
Focal seizure, or Todd's paralysis after a generalized seizure.
Migraine.
Hypoglycemia.
Intracranial mass lesion (tumor or abscess).

Prognosis
Of patients presenting with a TIA, 8% will have a stroke within the first week, and 10% within 90 days.
Higher risk of subsequent stroke in patients >age 60, with symptom duration longer than 10 minutes, or with history of diabetes.

Admit patients with new TIAs to a telemetry floor

Obtain an electrocardiogram, complete blood cell count, and coagulation profile

Perform computed tomography (CT) scan or magnetic resonance imaging (MRI) of the head to exclude stroke or intracranial hemorrhage
MRI is more sensitive than CT for identifying a stroke, especially in the first 24 hours. MRI reveals ischemic changes in ~50% of patients with TIA.

Start antiplatelet and anticoagulant therapy
Start all patients with a TIA on antiplatelet therapy with aspirin (75 to 325 mg/day) to reduce the risk of subsequent cerebrovascular event.
Patients with aspirin allergy should be treated with clopidogrel 75 mg/day.
Combined treatment with aspirin and clopidogrel may have greater benefit.
Start anticoagulation with heparin (and transition to warfarin) in patients with cardioembolic TIAs or TIAs from aortic atheromatous disease.

Aggressively treat modifiable risk factors
Smoking cessation; control of diabetes, hyperlipidemia, and hypertension.

Obtain a carotid ultrasound or MR angiography (MRA) to evaluate for carotid stenosis

Consider obtaining a transthoracic echocardiogram (TTE)
Evaluate for cardiac sources of emboli in patients without carotid vascular disease.
Should include a "bubble study" to evaluate for an atrial septal defect or patent foramen ovale.
Transesophageal echocardiography is more sensitive for identifying potential cardiac sources of emboli and should be performed if the TTE is unrevealing.

Consider obtaining a vascular surgery consult
Carotid endarterectomy should be performed in patients with TIAs and internal carotid artery stenosis of >70%, and should be considered if stenosis is 50% to 70%.
 • Significantly reduces the risk of ipsilateral stroke or recurrent TIA.
Percutaneous angioplasty and stenting is an alternative to carotid endarterectomy, especially in patients with high risk of perioperative complication.

S **What are the patient's symptoms?**
Common symptoms include:
- Unilateral extremity weakness
- Numbness or paresthesias
- Dysarthria
- Facial droop
- Vertigo or ataxia
- Aphasia or agnosia
- Visual change
- Dysphagia
- Mental status change

Headache and neck stiffness occur with intracranial or subarachnoid hemorrhage.
Classic posterior circulation symptoms include vertigo, ataxia, diplopia, deafness.
Classic anterior circulation symptoms include disorders of language and unilateral
    motor and sensory signs.
Deficits in multiple vascular territories suggest embolization from the heart or aorta.

What was the time course of the development of symptoms?
Embolic events are usually sudden in onset.
A stuttering course suggests atherosclerotic disease of the carotid or vertebral arteries.
Sudden severe headache suggests subarachnoid hemorrhage.
Headache progressing over minutes to hours suggests intracranial hemorrhage.

How long have the symptoms been present?
Patients who present within 3 hours of the onset of symptoms of an embolic stroke
    may be candidates for thrombolytic therapy (see below).
By definition, symptoms of a cerebrovascular accident (CVA) persist for greater than
    24 hours.

Does the patient have risk factors for vascular disease?
Risk factors for cerebrovascular disease are the same as for coronary artery disease:
- Diabetes mellitus
- Age (male
    >45 years; female
    >55 years)
- Hypertension
- Family history
    of premature
    coronary artery disease
- Dyslipidemia
- Smoking
- Other risk factors include homocystinemia, obesity, inactivity.

Does the patient have symptoms or a history of other vascular disease?
Cerebrovascular disease often coexists with coronary or peripheral vascular disease.

**Does the patient have conditions associated with thromboembolic
phenomena, hyperviscosity, or hypercoagulable syndromes?
(See SOAP 52 for list.)**

O **Perform a physical examination**
Vital signs:
- An irregular pulse may indicate atrial fibrillation.
- The presence of hypertension AND bradycardia may indicate increased
    intracranial pressure (Cushing's reflex).

Funduscopic examination: May reveal evidence of hypertensive retinopathy or
    "Hollenhorst" plaques (bright yellow cholesterol emboli).
Vascular examination: Listen carefully for carotid bruits.
Cardiac examination: Irregularly irregular rhythm suggests atrial fibrillation;
    regurgitant murmurs may suggest endocarditis; a S_3 suggests a cardiomyopathy.
Extremity examination: Look for evidence of peripheral embolization (digital
    ischemia) or manifestations of endocarditis (splinter hemorrhages, petechiae).
Neurologic examination: Should include assessment of mental status, speech, cranial
    nerves, strength, gait, reflexes, sensory exam, position and vibration sense.
- Serial neurologic examinations are essential to assess for progression or resolu-
    tion of symptoms.

Obtain an electrocardiogram
Look for arrhythmias that predispose to embolic events (e.g., afibrillation/flutter).

Ischemic cerebrovascular accident
The sudden loss of brain function caused by inadequate cerebral blood flow. Usually results from either atherosclerotic disease of the intracranial vessels; atheroembolic disease of the carotid or vertebral arteries, or the aorta; or thromboembolic disease from the heart (e.g., from atrial fibrillation, paradoxical emboli). Less commonly relates to hypotension-induced hypoperfusion.

Differential diagnosis
- Transient ischemic attack
- Migraine
- Seizure with post-ictal neurological deficit (Todd's paralysis)
- Intracranial hemorrhage
- Hypoglycemia

Obtain an emergent head computed tomography scan
Identify regions of cerebral infarction and exclude intracranial hemorrhage or mass. 60% of CT scans obtained within the first few hours after ischemic stroke are normal.

Assess stability of airway and the patient's breathing pattern
Patients with large CVAs may be unable to control their own airway and may require intubation and mechanical ventilation.

Admit to a monitored setting and obtain neurology consultation

Institute acute medical therapy
Consider thrombolytic therapy for patients presenting within 3 hours of symptom onset, who have no hemorrhage on head CT, and have no other contraindications.
- May reduce disability and death at 3 to 6 months but with an increased short-term risk of intracranial hemorrhage.
Start anticoagulation if the suspected mechanism of CVA is thromboembolism.
Start antiplatelet therapy (aspirin, clopidogrel) in patients with carotid artery disease.
Blood pressure (BP) should not be actively lowered in patients with an acute ischemic stroke unless the hypertension is extreme (i.e., systolic BP >180 mm Hg, diastolic BP >100 mm Hg).
- Normalization of BP acutely may precipitate cerebral hypoperfusion.
Control hyperthermia and hyperglycemia.
Deep venous thrombosis prophylaxis with low-molecular-eight heparin and/or lower extremity compression boots for all nonambulatory patients.

Obtain diagnostic studies to define etiology and extent of CVA
Obtain a carotid artery ultrasound or magnetic resonance imaging to evaluate for carotid arterial disease.
Obtain a transthoracic echocardiogram (TTE) to evaluate for embolic source.
- Perform a bubble study to exclude paradoxical embolism.
- Perform transesophageal echocardiography if TTE and carotid ultrasound unrevealing.
Perform magnetic resonance imaging (or repeat head CT in 24 to 48 hours) if initial study was normal.

Institute chronic medical therapy
Continue antiplatelet therapy (aspirin or clopidogrel) in patients with carotid disease.
Anticoagulate with warfarin in patients with cardioembolic disease.

Initiate aggressive risk factor modification in all patients with CVA
- Smoking cessation
- Lipid lowering
- Control of hypertension and diabetes

Obtain physical and occupational therapy consultation

S Does the patient have symptoms associated with pulmonary hypertension (PHTN)?

- Dyspnea on exertion   - Fatigue   - Chest pain   - Exertional syncope

Does the patient have symptoms associated with right heart failure?

- Edema   - Anorexia   - Increasing abdominal girth   - Abdominal pain

Does the patient have a condition that is associated with the development of PHTN?

- Chronic obstructive pulmonary disease
- Obstructive sleep apnea
- Mitral valve disease
- Pulmonary emboli
- Chronic anemia
- Cirrhosis
- Interstitial lung disease
- Left ventricular dysfunction
- Intracardiac shunts (atrial septal defect, ventricular septal defect, patent ductus arteriosus)
- Connective tissue disease (scleroderma, systemic lupus erythematosus)
- HIV
- Prior use of anorexigenic drugs (e.g., Phen-fen)

O Review vital signs

Tachypnea and decreased oxygen saturation may be noted (at rest or with exertion).

Perform a physical examination focusing on the following

Cardiac examination:

- A loud and often palpable pulmonic component of the second sound (P_2).
- A murmur of tricuspid regurgitation (TR).
- A right-sided S_4 (RVH) or S_3 (RV failure).
- A right ventricular heave.
- Elevated JVP; prominent V wave with tricuspid regurgitation.

Pulmonary examination:

- Wheezes (chronic obstructive pulmonary disease [COPD]).
- Rales (congestive heart failure).
- Fine crackles (interstitial fibrosis).

Abdominal examination:

- Hepatomegaly.
- Ascites.
- Pulsatile liver (with TR).

Review the patient's electrocardiogram

"Right sided strain pattern" (S1Q3T3), right atrial enlargement, right ventricular hypertrophy, right axis deviation, incomplete or complete right bundle branch block.

Review the patient's chest radiograph

Classically shows dilated central pulmonary arteries and pruning of peripheral vessels.
May show evidence of COPD, interstitial fibrosis, or bronchiectasis.
Loss of retrosternal air space on lateral film indicates right ventricular enlargement.

A Pulmonary hypertension

Defined as a systolic pressure of >25 mm Hg at rest or >30 mm Hg with exercise.
Divided into primary PHTN (no identifiable cause) and secondary PHTN.

Causes of secondary PHTN

Increased pulmonary artery blood flow (intra- and extra-cardiac shunts).
Pulmonary venous hypertension (left ventricular systolic or diastolic failure, MV disease).
Hypoxic pulmonary vasoconstriction (COPD, sleep apnea).
Reduction in pulmonary vasculature (pulmonary emboli, COPD, vasculitis).

Differential diagnosis
    - Angina   - Congestive heart failure   - Valvular heart disease
    - COPD or interstitial lung disease without pulmonary hypertension

P

Obtain a transthoracic echocardiograph
Can accurately estimate the pulmonary artery systolic pressure from the velocity of the tricuspid regurgitant jet (pressure = $4 \times$ velocity^2).
Evidence of RV pressure overload can be seen including RVH, RV dilatation, flattening of the interventricular septum, and a dilated inferior vena cava.

Consider right heart catheterization (Swan Ganz catheterization)
Allows for direct measurement of PA pressure and calculation of pulmonary vascular resistance (PVR).
- Can be measured serially to assess the effectiveness of medications.

Measure pulmonary capillary wedge pressure to exclude CHF as the cause of PHTN.

Obtain specific tests to evaluate for an underlying cause of pulmonary hypertension
High-resolution chest CT scan to evaluate for emphysema or pulmonary fibrosis.
Ventilation-perfusion scanning, CT-pulmonary angiography, and/or lower extremity ultrasound to evaluate for evidence of chronic thromboembolic disease.
Pulmonary function tests to evaluate for COPD.
Polysomnography ("sleep study") to evaluate for obstructive sleep apnea.
Liver function tests, HIV antibodies, and markers of connective tissue disease (ANA).

Start diuretic therapy for patients with right heart failure

Give supplemental oxygen for patients with hypoxemia

Start vasodilator therapy for patients with primary pulmonary hypertension
Continuous intravenous infusion of the prostacyclin analogue epoprostenol (Flolan).
- The most effective agent in the treatment of PHTN.
- Results in improvement in clinical symptoms and a reduction in mortality in patients with NYHA class III–IV heart failure symptoms.
- Newer agents such as the subcutaneous prostacyclin analogue treprostinil and an inhaled analog iloprost (inhaled six to nine times/day) are being investigated.

Oral calcium channel blockers such as nifedipine or diltiazem.
- Result in improvement in ~25% of patients.

Oral endothelin receptor antagonists such as bosentan.
Phosphodiesterase inhibitors such as cilostazol (a drug primarily indicated for claudication) and sildenafil (an agent primarily indicated for erectile dysfunction) may be of benefit in some patients.

Treat the underlying cause of secondary PHTN
Bronchodilators and oxygen for COPD.
Nocturnal continuous positive airway pressure (CPAP) mask for sleep apnea.
Routine treatment for congestive heart failure. (See SOAP 11.)
Consider closure of intracardiac shunts (ASD, VSD, PDA).
- May not be feasible in patients with severe PHTN and right heart failure.

Start anticoagulation for chronic pulmonary thromboembolic disease.
- Surgical thrombectomy should be considered for large, central PEs.

Consider starting vasodilator therapy.
- May be less effective than for primary PHTN.

Consider lung or heart-lung transplantation in patients with refractory symptoms despite maximal medical therapy

S **What are the patient's current symptoms?**

Most patients present with ischemic symptoms in their extremities.
- Claudication of the hands, arms, legs, or feet
- Ischemic digital ulcerations (present in two thirds of patients)

Symptoms may be intermittent with quiescent periods of weeks to years.

Does the patient have Raynaud's phenomena?
- Sequential white, blue, red color changes of the digits on exposure to cold and rewarming.
- Occurs commonly with thromboangiitis obliterans (TAO), but is not specific.

May present with a triad of Raynaud's phenomenon, claudication, and migratory superficial thrombophlebitis.

How many cigarettes does the patient smoke?
A history of smoking is almost universally present in patients with TAO.

May occur with use of smokeless tobacco.

Is the patient in a demographic group in which TAO commonly occurs?
Usually occurs in young, male smokers who are between 40 and 45 years of age.

Highest incidence of TAO occurs in the Middle East, Far East, and Eastern Europe (especially among those of Ashkenazi Jewish ancestry).

Increased incidence in patients with HLA-B5 and HLA-A9.

O **Perform a thorough vascular examination looking for**

Localized ischemia or ulceration of distal extremities; may be asymmetric.
- A single digit or an entire foot/hand may be pale or cold.

Rubor, especially when the limb is dependent.

Evidence of superficial thrombophlebitis.

Findings suspicious for TAO in a symptomatic extremity should prompt a thorough examination of other (asymptomatic) extremities.

Examine for evidence of other underlying diseases that may present with similar peripheral findings
Malar or discoid rash of lupus.

Cutaneous abnormalities of scleroderma.

Arthritic changes of rheumatoid disease.

Evidence of atherosclerotic vascular disease (e.g., carotid or femoral bruits).

A **Thromboangiitis obliterans (Buerger's disease)**
A nonatherosclerotic inflammatory disease of the small and medium-sized arteries and veins of the arms and legs.
- Occasionally involves the coronary, cerebral, renal, and mesenteric vessels.
- Inflammatory thrombi occlude arteries and veins.
- Results in acquired endothelial dysfunction.

Differential diagnosis
- Systemic embolization
- Systemic lupus erythematosus
- Rheumatoid arthritis (vasculitis)
- Hypercoagulable states
- Scleroderma or CREST syndrome
- Other vasculitides

P **Check serum inflammatory markers**
There are no specific laboratory markers for TAO.
- Erythrocyte sedimentation rate (ESR), C-reactive protein (CRP), antinuclear antibodies (ANA), and rheumatoid factor (RF) are normal with TAO.

Perform laboratory tests to exclude alternate diagnoses
Vasculitis: Check ANA, ESR, and RF.
Lupus: Check anti–double-stranded DNA.
Hypercoagulable state: Check antiphospholipid antibody, homocysteine level, protein S, and protein C.
Scleroderma: Check anti-centromere antibody.

Obtain an echocardiogram to exclude cardioembolic disease

Obtain angiograms of all four limbs
Characteristic findings include:
- Segmental occlusion of the distal aspect of small and medium-sized vessels in the extremities.
- "Corkscrew collateralization" around areas of occlusion.
Disease is almost always infrapopliteal in the legs and distal to the brachial artery in the arms.

Consider biopsy if diagnosis uncertain (rarely necessary)
With active disease an intravascular, occlusive, highly cellular, inflammatory thrombus is seen with relative sparing of vessel walls.

Mandate SMOKING CESSATION
This is the most effective therapy for TAO.
Significantly reduces the need for amputation, which occurs in:
- 6% of patients who stop smoking.
- 57% of patients who continue to smoke.

Institute medical therapy
Aspirin (81–325 mg daily) is used empirically.
Iloprost (an IV prostaglandin analog) may reduce the need for amputation.
- Usually reserved for patients with critical limb ischemia, during the initial period of smoking cessation.
Surgical revascularization is not useful because of the diffuse nature of the disease and the distal location of the vascular involvement.

S **Does the patient have symptoms attributable to an atrial myxoma?**
Approximately 10% of patients with myxomas are asymptomatic.

Does the patient have nonspecific systemic symptoms?
Patients with myxomas commonly report fever, malaise, weight loss, arthralgias, and
Raynaud's phenomena.

Does the patient have symptoms of mitral or tricuspid valve disease?
Left atrial myxomas may obstruct the mitral valve and mimic mitral stenosis:
  • Dyspnea on exertion   • Acute pulmonary edema
  • Paroxysmal nocturnal dyspnea • Exertional syncope
Symptoms are often positional—the tumor may obstruct the valve only when the
patient is in the upright position.
Right atrial myxomas occasionally obstruct the tricuspid valve and produce symptoms
of right heart failure:
      • Fatigue   • Edema   • Dyspnea

Does the patient have symptoms of embolic phenomenon?
Left-sided myxomas can cause systemic emboli to cerebral, coronary, mesenteric,
renal, or peripheral arteries resulting in stroke, myocardial infarction, abdominal
ischemia, or limb ischemia.
Right-sided myxomas can cause recurrent pulmonary emboli.
  • Paradoxical emboli can occur in the presence of an intracardiac shunt.

Obtain a thorough review of systems

Obtain a family history
Although most myxomas are sporadic, they can occur in an autosomal dominant
pattern as part of the Carney complex.
  • Multiple nevi, extracardiac myxoid tumors, endocrine overactivity, melanotic
    schwannoma, and multiple cardiac myxomas.

 Check vital signs
Patients with myxoma may have fever and may develop atrial fibrillation.

Perform a thorough cardiovascular examination
May hear a low-pitched diastolic murmur similar to that of mitral stenosis.
  • Results from obstruction of the mitral valve by the tumor ("pseudo mitral
    stenosis").
Tumor plop: diastolic sound related to prolapse of the tumor across the mitral valve.
A loud P_2 indicates pulmonary hypertension.
A murmur of mitral regurgitation is less common.

Perform a skin and extremity examination
Look for evidence of distal embolization.
Cutaneous myxomas and multiple pigmented nevi may be present in familial cases.

Review the patient's electrocardiogram
Left atrial enlargement is the most common finding.
Other findings include atrial fibrillation or flutter, right ventricular hypertrophy.

Review laboratory results
Myxomas are often associated with anemia, elevated erythrocyte sedimentation rate,
elevated C-reactive protein.

Atrial myxoma

Atrial myxomas are the most common primary tumor of the heart. Although benign histologically, they can cause valvular obstruction or distal embolization. Seventy-five percent arise in the left atrium (usually at the site of the fossa ovalis). Right atrial and left ventricular tumors are less common. They are multifocal in 5% of cases.

Differential diagnosis

Symptoms may mimic those of mitral stenosis, vasculitis, atheroembolic disease, or collagen vascular disease.
Echocardiographic features must be distinguished from:
- Other cardiac tumors
- Intracardiac thrombus
- Endocarditis

 Obtain an echocardiogram

Confirms the presence of an intracardiac mass.
Evaluate for dysfunction of the mitral valve or tricuspid valve.
Evaluate the structure of the tumor:
- Polypoid tumors have much greater propensity to both embolize and prolapse into the ventricle than do sessile tumors.

Transesophageal echocardiography produces superior images and may be required to confirm the diagnosis if the results of the transthoracic echocardiogram are not definitive.

Consider cardiac magnetic resonance imaging if the diagnosis is in doubt

Can better define the anatomy of the tumor and identify myocardial invasion.
Can better differentiate between tumor and thrombus.

Obtain a cardiothoracic surgical consult

Consider tumor resection

Usually curative with low risk of recurrence in sporadic cases.
- Lesions may recur as a result of incomplete excision, growth of a secondary tumor implant, or development of a new primary lesion in a patient with a familial myxoma syndrome.

Biannual echocardiography is indicated to screen for recurrence for at least 5 years after resection.

S What kind of injury has the patient suffered?

Cardiac contusion is almost always associated with blunt chest trauma.

~75% of patients with cardiac contusion have obvious evidence of other injuries.

Common associated thoracic injuries include:

- Rib fractures
- Lung contusion
- Sternal fracture
- Pneumothorax
- Clavicular fracture
- Chest wall hematoma

What are the patient's symptoms?

May be asymptomatic or masked by symptoms of other injuries.

Symptoms specific to cardiac contusion are varied.

- Chest/precordial pain is the most common symptom—may be due to chest wall injury but can be myocardial or pericardial in origin.

Palpitations and syncope

- Premature atrial or ventricular beats are common.
- High degree atrioventricular (AV) block, supraventricular and ventricular arrhythmias can occur.

Symptoms of congestive heart failure:

- Acutely due to myocardial injury, mitral valve/papillary muscle rupture, or pericardial tamponade.
- Chronically due to dilated cardiomyopathy following myocardial injury.

Hemodynamic collapse or sudden death may result from:

- Ventricular rupture.
- *Commotio Cordis*—blunt chest trauma during the repolarization phase of the cardiac cycle may result in ventricular arrhythmias and sudden cardiac death.

- After severe trauma, hemodynamic instability is more likely to be due to non-cardiac injury (i.e., hypovolemia, pulmonary, neurologic, or vascular injury).

O Check vital signs

Tachycardia and hypotension are commonly present.

Perform a cardiac examination looking especially for

Elevated jugular venous pressure and muffled heart sounds suggestive of tamponade.

Pericardial friction rub.

An S_3 or S_4 suggestive of heart failure.

A holosystolic murmur of tricuspid or mitral regurgitation.

Look for evidence of other traumatic injuries

Review the chest radiograph

May identify thoracic trauma as well as evidence of a large pericardial effusion.

Obtain a 12-lead electrocardiogram

Features are varied and nonspecific:

- Sinus tachycardia
- Diffuse or regional ST elevations
- Right bundle branch block
- Ventricular or supraventricular arrhythmias
- Atrial or ventricular ectopy
- Q-waves
- Fascicular or AV blocks
- Prolonged Q-T interval

Obtain cardiac enzyme levels

Creatine kinase is elevated after muscle trauma and of minimal diagnostic utility for cardiac contusion. MB isoforms are more specific.

Troponin I and T are more cardiac specific and predictive of cardiac injury.

Cardiac contusion
Myocardial injury caused by blunt chest trauma, usually associated with motor vehicle accidents. Injury is due to compression of the heart between the sternum and spine or a deceleration injury with the right ventricle (RV) impacting the sternum. The RV is most frequently injured, although the interventricular septum and left ventricular (LV) apex may also be involved.

Incidence
Of those with significant blunt chest trauma, 15% to 25% will have evidence of cardiac injury by biochemical assay (troponin) and up to 50% on electrocardiography (ECG) or echocardiography.

Differential diagnosis
- Cardiac ischemia	- Pericardial tamponade	- Aortic dissection
- Pneumothorax	- Pulmonary artery injury	- Sternum/rib fracture
- Fat embolism	- Pulmonary contusion	

 Admit to a monitored setting

Triage patient based on severity of thoracic injury
If minimal injury, hemodynamically stable, and with normal ECG and normal troponin, most patients can be safely discharged within 24 hours.
If enzyme levels become positive or ECG changes develop, patient should be monitored for 24 to 48 hours.
If hemodynamically unstable or hemodynamically stable but with severe thoracic injuries (i.e., sternal fracture, multiple rib fractures, lung contusion), admit to an intensive care unit.

Obtain an echocardiogram
Evaluate extent of myocardial damage.
Assess presence and significance of pericardial effusion.
Exclude associated acute valvular dysfunction.
Transesophageal echocardiogram may be necessary in patients in whom transthoracic images are limited as a result of extensive chest wall injury.

Avoid anticoagulation
May precipitate or exacerbate intramyocardial or pericardial hemorrhage.

Administer analgesia (opiates) for pain control
Avoid nonsteroidal anti-inflammatory drugs because these may interfere with myocardial healing.

Treat associated injuries

Institute long-term therapy once the patient is hemodynamically stable
Treatment is similar to that for myocardial infarction.
- Angiotensin-converting enzyme inhibitors and beta-blockers for LV dysfunction/heart failure.
- Cardiac rehabilitation after recovery from trauma.
- Antiplatelet agents are not required in the absence of associated coronary artery disease.

S **Does the patient have any symptoms of hypercholesterolemia?**
Most patients have no specific signs or symptoms of high cholesterol levels.
Rarely, very high levels of triglycerides can cause pancreatitis.

Does the patient have any symptoms related to cardiovascular or cerebrovascular disease?

- Angina
- Claudication
- Cerebrovascular accident/transient ischemic attack
- Intestinal angina

Elevated cholesterol is closely associated with vascular disease.

Does the patient have any condition that predisposes to developing hyperlipidemia?

- Hypothyroidism
- Alcohol abuse
- Type II diabetes
- Obesity
- Nephrotic syndrome
- High fat diet

Does the patient have other risk factors for coronary artery disease?

- Diabetes mellitus
- High-density lipoprotein (HDL) <35 mg/dL
- Family history of premature CAD (male <55 yrs; female <60 yrs)
- Hypertension
- Age (male >45 years; female >55 years)
- Cigarette smoking

- 50% to 70% of families with premature coronary artery disease (CAD) will have a familial hyperlipidemia.

Review medications
Corticosteroids and progestins can elevate cholesterol.
Diuretics, beta-blockers, estrogens can elevate triglycerides.

O **Review vital signs**

Perform a directed physical examination
Funduscopic examination:
- Hypertensive retinopathy.
- Lipemia retinalis (milky white retinal vessels) due to elevated triglycerides.
Vascular examination:
- Listen for bruits in the carotid, vertebral, subclavian, and femoral arteries.
- A bruit indicates turbulent flow through a diseased artery.
- Feel for enlargement of the abdominal aorta and listen for abdominal bruits.
Cardiac examination:
- Listen for an aortic sclerotic or stenotic murmur (may radiate to the carotids).
Extremity examination:
- Look for evidence of pulmonary artery disease as well as eruptive or tendinous xanthoma.
Skin examination:
- Look for xanthelasma (yellowish plaques around the eyes).

Obtain a fasting lipid panel, including total cholesterol (TC), HDL, and triglycerides (TG)
A calculation of low-density lipoprotein (LDL) can be made (LDL = TC − (HDL + TG/5)).
This calculation is inaccurate if the triglycerides are >400.
- Note that acute stress (such as a myocardial infarction [MI]) may falsely lower LDL for up to 2 months.

Exclude causes of secondary hypercholesterolemia
Check thyroid-stimulating hormone, fasting glucose, hemoglobin A1C, and renal function.

A **Hyperlipidemia**
A group of disorders characterized by abnormally elevated serum levels of lipoproteins and associated with the development of atherosclerotic vascular disease.

Etiology
Usually multifactorial (dietary factors, obesity, inactivity, genetic predisposition). Purely genetic causes account for a minority of cases.
- Genetic defects result in altered metabolism of lipoproteins.

Secondary causes of hyperlipidemia include hypothyroidism, nephrotic syndrome, type II diabetes, alcoholism, obesity, and certain medications (see previous section).

P **Instruct on therapeutic lifestyle changes**   <AQ: 30
Low fat diet (<7% of total calories from saturated fat; <200 mg cholesterol/day).   minutes?>
Weight loss in overweight patients.
Aerobic exercise (>30 minutes at least four times a week).
Control of diabetes and hypertension.

Perform a risk assessment to determine whether the patient is an appropriate candidate for drug therapy (see Table 58-1). Important considerations include
LDL level.
Presence of CAD (angina, MI, abnormal stress test, CAD on angiography).
Presence of CAD equivalents (diabetes, peripheral vascular disease).
Number of CAD risk factors (smoking, low HDL, hypertension, family history of premature CAD, age [male >45 years; female >55 years]).

Initiate lipid-lowering therapy to attain goal LDL based on risk category (see Table 58-1)
HMG Co-A reductase inhibitors are first-line therapy for elevated LDL.
- Atorvastatin, lovastatin, pravastatin, simvastatin, rosuvastatin.
- Most potent drugs for decreasing LDL (20% to 60% LDL lowering).
- Modest HDL increasing (5%) and triglyceride decreasing (20%) effects.

If goal LDL is not achieved with statin therapy, use combination therapy with:
- Ezetimibe (a cholesterol absorption inhibitor)—reduces LDL an additional 14%.
- Fibrates (gemfibrozil, fenofibrate) lower TG (35% to 50%) and increase HDL (15% to 25%).
- Nicotinic acid (niacin)—lowers TG and LDL cholesterol and increases HDL.
- Bile acid sequestrants (cholestyramine, colestipol)—lower LDL ~25%.

Fibrates are first-line therapy for isolated elevation in triglycerides.

Check liver function test results before initiation of drug therapy

Check fasting lipid panel and liver function test results 6 to 12 weeks after starting therapy or changing dose

Table 58-1 Risk Assessment		
Risk Category	**LDL Goal (mg/dL)**	**LDL Level to Start Drug Therapy**
CAD or CAD risk equivalent	<100	≥130 (100–129: drug optional)
No CAD with ≥2 risk factors	<130	≥160
No CAD and 0–1 risk factors	<160	≥190 (160–190: drug optional)
Very high risk (recent MI; CAD + DM; metabolic syndrome)	<70	>100 (70–100: drug optional)

CAD = Coronary artery disease; DM = diabetes mellitus; LDL = low-density lipoprotein; MI = myocardial infarction.

S **Does the patient have any symptoms?**

Most patients have no specific signs or symptoms of an elevated C-reactive protein (CRP).

Does the patient have symptoms related to cardiovascular or cerebrovascular disease?

- An elevated CRP in patients with vascular disease is associated with a worse prognosis.
- Elevated CRP may correlate with disease activity.

Does the patient have any symptoms or conditions that may elevate CRP?

Any inflammatory condition may be associated with an elevated CRP:

- Chronic inflammatory diseases (e.g., rheumatoid arthritis, vasculitis)
- Major infection
- Neoplasm
- Trauma

Does the patient have other risk factors for vascular disease?

- Diabetes mellitus   - Hypertension   - Cigarette smoking
- Hyperlipidemia   - Age (male >45 years; female >55 years)
- Family history of premature coronary artery disease (CAD)
  (male <55 years; female <60 years)

Elevated CRP enhances the risk associated with these established cardiovascular risk factors.

O **Review vital signs**

Perform a directed physical examination looking for evidence of vascular disease

Funduscopic examination:
- Hypertensive retinopathy.

Vascular examination:
- Listen for bruits in the carotid, vertebral, subclavian, and femoral arteries.
- Feel for enlargement of the abdominal aorta and listen for abdominal bruits.

Cardiac examination:
- Listen for an aortic valve murmur.
- Assess for evidence of a cardiomyopathy or heart failure.

Extremity examination:
- Look for evidence of peripheral vascular disease.
- Look for cutaneous manifestations of hyperlipidemia (e.g., eruptive or tendinous xanthoma).

Obtain a fasting lipid panel including total cholesterol (TC), high-density lipoproteins (HDL), and triglycerides (TG)

The low-density lipoprotein (LDL) level can be calculated (LDL = TC − (HDL + TG/5)).

- Note that acute stress (such as an MI or infection) may transiently lower LDL and increase CRP.

A **Elevated C-reactive protein**
CRP is a nonspecific marker for inflammation that has been shown to predict cardiovascular risk in asymptomatic patients and has prognostic implications in patients with cardiovascular disease.
- It is uncertain if CRP is simply a marker of inflammation or has a pathophysiologic role in atherosclerosis.
- It remains uncertain if lowering CRP reduces the risk of cardiovascular disease.
- The odds ratio of a patient with an elevated CRP developing coronary heart disease is 1.5:1 (i.e., a 50% increased risk).

Classification of CRP level
Low risk: <1 mg/L
Intermediate risk: 1 to 3 mg/L
High risk: >3 mg/L

Recommendations for the use of CRP
Consider checking as part of a risk assessment panel in patients without established cardiovascular disease but with an intermediate Framingham risk score (10% to 20% 10-year risk of coronary heart disease).
- Patients with an elevated CRP need further assessment of risk factors.
- May have a lower threshold to treat other risk factors in patients with elevated CRP.

CRP should not be used to determine the type or aggressiveness of therapy in patients with established cardiovascular disease.

P **Perform a risk factor assessment (once an elevated CRP is identified)**
Calculate 10-year risk for developing coronary heart disease (Framingham Risk Score). As a tool for risk stratification, CRP is most useful in the intermediate risk patient to encourage more aggressive risk reduction therapy.

Aggressively manage established risk factors, especially in moderate- and high-risk patients

- Cholesterol reduction	- Smoking cessation	- Blood pressure control
- Glycemic control	- Weight loss in overweight individuals	

Counsel all patients regarding a healthy diet and an exercise regimen

Consider further evaluation for "evolving" risk factors
Hypertriglyceridemia:
- May be an independent risk factor for CAD.
Lipoprotein(a):
- A modified LDL with anti-fibrinolytic properties.
Apolipoprotein analysis:
- Elevated apolipoprotein B-100 and low apolipoprotein A-1 may better represent LDL and HDL levels, respectively.

Consider specific therapy to lower CRP (not indicated independent of other risk factors)
HMG Co-A reducatase inhibitors (statins) and beta-blockers appear to lower CRP levels.
Estrogen replacement therapy elevates CRP levels.
Aspirin has no effect on CRP levels.

S **Does the patient have symptoms related to cardiovascular or cerebrovascular disease?**

- Angina pectoris   - Transient ischemic attack
- Claudication   - Heart failure

Elevated homocysteine levels are associated with an increased risk of vascular disease, especially in patients with few other risk factors.

Does the patient have other established risk factors for vascular disease?

- Diabetes mellitus   - Hypertension
- Hyperlipidemia   - Age (male >45 years;
- Family history of   female >55 years)
  premature coronary   - Cigarette smoking
  artery disease (CAD)
  (male <55 years;
  female <60 years)

Hyperhomocystinemia is not as strong a risk factor as other cardiovascular risk factors.

Does the patient have a history of deep venous thrombosis or pulmonary embolism?

Hyperhomocystinemia is associated with a 2.5- to threefold increase in the risk of thromboembolic disease.

If the patient is female, does she have a history of obstetrical complications?

Hyperhomocystinemia is associated with an increased risk of preeclampsia, abruptio placentae, fetal growth retardation, and stillbirth.

Does the patient have a family history of premature CAD or thromboembolic disease?

Take a dietary history

Does the patient eat green leafy vegetables (source of folate) and dairy products (source of vitamin B12)?

Homocysteine levels are inversely proportional to folate, and vitamin B6 and B12 intake.

Obtain a medical history

Does the patient have premature coronary, cerebral, or peripheral vascular disease?

Macrocytic anemia may result from vitamin B12 or folate deficiency.

Autoimmune diseases and surgical gastrectomy may result in pernicious anemia (vitamin B12 deficiency).

 Review vital signs

Perform a directed physical examination

Vascular examination:
- Listen for bruits in the carotid, vertebral, subclavian and femoral arteries.
- Feel for enlargement of the abdominal aorta and listen for abdominal bruits.

Extremity examination:
- Look for evidence of peripheral vascular disease (shiny, hairless skin; digital ischemia).

Review fasting lipid panel

Total cholesterol (TC), high-density lipoprotein (HDL), and triglycerides (TG) are measured directly.

Calculate LDL (LDL = TC − (HDL + TG/5).

Review the patient's ECG for evidence of ischemic heart disease

Hyperhomocystinemia

Homocysteine is an amino acid that is formed by the conversion of methionine to cysteine. It displays both atherogenic and prothrombotic properties and, when elevated, is an independent risk factor for atherosclerotic vascular disease and venous thromboembolic disease. Mild to moderately elevated homocysteine has been identified in 5% to 7% of the general population.

Classification of serum homocysteine levels
Normal: 5 to 15 μmol/L.
Mildly elevated: 16 to 30 μmol/L.
Moderately elevated: 30 to 100 μmol/L.
Severely elevated: >100 μmol/L.

 Check serum homocysteine level in patients with the following conditions

Premature vascular disease, especially if there are no other significant risk factors.
Unexplained or recurrent venous thrombosis.

Check serum levels of vitamin B12 and folate levels
B vitamin deficiency may be responsible for 2/3 of cases of hyperhomocysteinemia.

Start dietary modification in all patients with elevated serum homocysteine levels
Encourage a diet high in fruits, vegetables, and low-fat dairy products.
Avoid saturated fats.

Institute pharmacologic therapy in all patients with severely elevated homocysteine and in patients with CAD or venous thrombosis and even mildly elevated homocysteine
Start pharmacologic therapy with:
- Folate: 1 to 5 mg daily (alone or combined with the vitamins below).
  - The dose of folate should be increased from 1 to 5 mg daily to achieve a homocysteine level of <15 μmol/L.
  - Homocysteine levels usually normalize within 2–6 weeks of starting therapy.
- Pyridoxine (vitamin B6): 10 mg daily.
- Cobalamin (vitamin B12): 0.4 mg (orally) daily.
  - Given to prevent neuropathy associated with vitamin B12 deficiency.
- There is still no conclusive evidence that lowering homocysteine results in improved cardiovascular outcomes.

Consider withholding treatment for 6 months after percutaneous coronary revascularization, as B-complex vitamins appear to increase the risk of stent restenosis.

Aggressively manage risk factors, especially in moderate- and high-risk patients
Diet and exercise counseling in all patients.
Lipid-lowering therapy based on current guidelines.
Smoking cessation.
Blood pressure control.
Glycemic control in diabetics.

S **Why did the patient have the coronary calcium score (CCS) performed?**
Screening for coronary artery disease (CAD): Assessment of CCS in asymptomatic patients may identify CAD at an earlier point in time.
Further risk stratification: Assessment of CCS in patients at moderate risk for CAD may identify those who have a higher than suspected risk.

Does the patient have any symptoms of coronary artery disease?
Coronary artery calcification is a marker of coronary atherosclerosis.
The role of CCS in patients with established CAD is not well defined.

Does the patient have other established risk factors for coronary vascular disease?

- Diabetes mellitus   - Hypertension   - Cigarette smoking
- Hyperlipidemia   - Age (male >45 years;
                             female >55 years)
- Family history of premature CAD (male <55 years; female <60 years)

These factors can be used to calculate the 10-year risk of cardiac event based on the Framingham risk score.

What was the result of the coronary calcium score?
The CCS reflects the quantity of calcium in the coronary arteries on computed tomography.
Scores range from 0 to greater than 400 and reflect incremental increases in the risk of CAD (see Table 61-1).

 Review vital signs

Perform a directed physical examination looking for evidence of vascular disease
Funduscopic examination:
  • Assess for hypertensive retinopathy.
Vascular examination:
  • Listen for bruits in the carotid, vertebral, subclavian, and femoral arteries.
  • Feel for enlargement of the abdominal aorta and listen for abdominal bruits.
Cardiac examination:
  • Listen for a systolic ejection murmur at the upper sternal border resulting from aortic valve sclerosis or stenosis. (See SOAP 24.)
Extremity examination:
  • Look for evidence of peripheral artery disease.
    ◆ Diminished distal pulses, loss of hair in the extremities, digital ischemia.
  • Look for eruptive or tendinous xanthoma indicative of hyperlipidemia.

Table 61-1	Coronary Calcium Score
0	Unlikely any plaque burden and very low cardiovascular risk.
1–10	Minimal plaque burden and low cardiovascular risk.
11–100	At least mild plaque burden with moderate cardiovascular risk.
101–400	Moderate plaque burden with moderately high cardiovascular risk.
>400	Extensive plaque burden with high likelihood of obstructive coronary artery disease and at high risk for cardiovascular event.

Review laboratories
Fasting lipid panel:
- Total cholesterol (TC), high-density lipoprotein (HDL), and triglycerides (TG) can be measured.
- Low-density lipoprotein (LDL) is calculated (LDL = TC – (HDL + TG/5)).
Fasting glucose and hemoglobin A1c level.

Coronary calcium score
Coronary calcification occurs as part of the atherosclerotic process; its extent can be measured noninvasively using electron beam CT (EBCT). The extent of coronary calcification correlates with the atherosclerotic burden, severity of CAD, and risk of future coronary vascular events.
- The sensitivity for a coronary stenosis >50% ranges from 90% to 100% while the specificity ranges from 45% to 76%.
- A CCS >200 in patients >50 years old, and >100 in those <50 years old correlates very strongly with the presence of obstructive CAD.
- A CCS of 0 strongly suggests the absence of CAD.

Current utility of CCS
CCS may be able to identify asymptomatic patients who are at increased risk for adverse cardiac events, but uncertain if this affects outcome.
CCS may provide independent prognostic information when compared to the Framingham risk score.
The greatest utility may be in the patient who is felt clinically to be at intermediate risk—CCS may identify both higher and lower risk groups among these patients.

Evolving roles for coronary calcium testing
Noninvasive differentiation of ischemic and nonischemic cardiomyopathy.
Identification of chest pain patients at low risk for cardiac morbidity or mortality.

Perform an extensive risk factor assessment
Quantify the Framingham risk score.
Apply the CCS to the clinical/Framingham risk score for further risk stratification.

Consider other cardiac testing for further risk stratification
In asymptomatic patients with a very low CCS (0–10):
- The risk of significant CAD is low.
- Further testing should be directed by development of clinical symptoms.
In asymptomatic patients with a moderate CCS (11–400):
- The risk of CAD is increased.
- Consider stress testing to further clarify cardiac risk.
In asymptomatic patients with high CCS (>400):
- The risk of CAD is high and further evaluation and management may be warranted.
- Consider further evaluation with noninvasive testing.
- No clear indication for cardiac catheterization in the absence of symptoms or objective evidence of ischemia.

Institute aggressive risk factor modification
Lipid lowering based on the NCEP guidelines. (See SOAP 58.)
Smoking cessation.
Hypertension control.
Glycemic control in diabetics.
Diet and exercise.

S

How was the diagnosis of left ventricular hypertrophy (LVH) made?
Usually noted incidentally on electrocardiography (ECG) or by echocardiography.

Does the patient have factors that predispose LVH?
Pressure overload states:
- Hypertension (most common cause of LVH).
- Aortic stenosis.
- Coarctation of the aorta.

Volume overload states:
- Aortic or mitral regurgitation.

Hypertrophic cardiomyopathy (HCM):
- A group of genetic diseases of the cardiac sarcomere characterized by hypertrophy of the left ventricle.

Perform a review of systems
Many patients with LVH are asymptomatic.
Dyspnea on exertion is common:
- LV thickening results in diastolic dysfunction.
- LV systolic dysfunction may occur with long-standing hypertension or advanced valvular heart disease.

Chest pain:
- May reflect decreased myocardial blood flow resulting from coronary artery disease and/or increased myocardial demand resulting from increased LV mass.

Palpitations are frequent:
- Left atrial enlargement predisposes to atrial arrhythmias.
- HCM and hypertensive cardiomyopathy may cause ventricular arrhythmias.

Other symptoms relate to the underlying disorder:
- Hypertension: headache, visual changes.
- Aortic stenosis: syncope.

O

Check vital signs
Check blood pressure in both arms.

Perform a physical examination
Funduscopic examination:
- Look for evidence of hypertensive retinopathy.

Cardiac examination:
- LV pressure overload results in an LV heave.
- The point of maximal impulse will be displaced laterally if there is LV dilation.
- An S_4 is usually present.
   ◆ Reflects atrial contraction into a poorly compliant LV.
- Listen for murmurs of aortic or mitral valve stenosis or regurgitation.

Review the patient's ECG
Common criteria for LVH include:
- Sum of S wave in V_1 and R wave in V_5 or V_6 >35 mm; *OR*
- Sum of S wave in V_2 and R wave in V_5 or V_6 >45 mm; *OR*
- Height of R wave in V_5 >26 mm; *OR*
- Height of R wave in lead I >14 mm; *OR*
- Height of R wave in aVL >11 mm (the most specific sign)

ECG is only 50% sensitive and 80% specific for LVH.
Other concomitant findings include:
- A "strain pattern" (ST segment depression and/or T-wave inversions in leads with tall R waves).

- Left axis deviation.
- Left atrial enlargement.

A **Left ventricular hypertrophy**

An increase in LV mass resulting from hypertrophy of existing myocytes.
- Usually a secondary response to pressure or volume overload.
  - ◆ Pressure overload results in concentric hypertrophy (a thickened LV).
  - ◆ Volume overload results in eccentric hypertrophy (a dilated LV).
- Occasionally reflects a primary myocardial abnormality (HCM).

Must be distinguished from infiltrative myocardial diseases (e.g., amyloidosis).
- These are characterized by LV thickening due to protein deposition, not myocyte hypertrophy.
- ECG in patients with infiltrative disease usually reveals low QRS voltage.

Prognosis

Patients with LVH have an increased risk of:
- Congestive heart failure
- Cerebrovascular events
- Death after MI
- Atrial fibrillation
- Sudden cardiac death due to arrhythmia

P **Consider echocardiography**

Criteria for LVH on echocardiogram include:
- LV mass >124 g/m^2.
- LV wall thickness >11 mm.

In patients with borderline hypertension, the presence of LVH is an indication for medical therapy.

Evaluate for valvular dysfunction (aortic stenosis, aortic insufficiency, mitral regurgitation) contributing to pressure or volume overload.

Assess for evidence of HCM.

Aggressively treat hypertension

Sodium restriction, dietary modification, exercise, and weight loss have been shown to promote regression of LVH.

Antihypertensive agents reduce LVH by lowering blood pressure and via promoting reverse LV remodeling (LVH regression).
- Angiotensin receptor blockers, calcium channel blockers, and ACE inhibitors may induce more regression of LVH than beta-blockers or direct-acting vasodilator agents.

Assess and treat other underlying conditions

Index

A

Adenosine
  for stress testing, 21
  in Wolff-Parkinson-White syndrome, 85
  in AVNRT, 87
Amiodarone, in ventricular tachycardia, 89
  in atrial fibrillation, 79
Angina, 2–3
  Prinzmetal's (variant), 12–13
  stable, 14–15
  unstable, 16–17
Angiography
  in cardiogenic shock, 35
  in carotid bruit, 103
  in thromboangiitis obliterans, 111
Angiotensin-converting enzyme (ACE)
  inhibitors
  in dilated cardiomyopathy, 31
  in hypertension, 91
  in mitral regurgitation, 51
  in myocardial infarction, 19
  in systolic heart failure, 23
Ankle brachial index, 99
Antibiotics, in endocarditis, 57
Anticoagulants
  in atrial fibrillation, 79
  in atrial flutter, 81
  in cerebrovascular accident, 107
  in transient ischemic attack, 105
Anti-hypertensive therapy, 91
Antiplatelet therapy
  in cerebrovascular accident, 107
  in myocardial infarction, 17, 19
  in peripheral arterial disease, 99
  in transient ischemic attack, 105
Aortic coarctation, 100–101
Aortic dissection, 2, 41, 96–97
Aortic insufficiency, 52–53
Aortic stenosis, 48–49
Aortic valve, bicuspid, 62–63
Aortography, in aortic coarctation, 101
Arrhythmias. *See also specific arrhythmias*
  atrial, 78–81
  supraventricular, 8
  ventricular, 88–89
  in Wolff-Parkinson-White syndrome,
    84–85

Arterial disease, peripheral, 98–99
Aspirin
  in carotid bruit, 103
  in myocardial infarction, 17
  in stable angina, 15
  in thromboangiitis obliterans, 111
Atrial fibrillation, 78–79
Atrial flutter, 80–81
Atrial myxoma, 112–113
Atrial septal defect, 60–61
Atrioventricular nodal reentrant
  tachycardia, 86–87
Atropine, in complete heart block, 75
Austin-Flint murmur, 52

B

Balloon valvuloplasty
  in mitral stenosis, 47
  in pulmonary stenosis, 65
Beck's triad, 40
Beta-blockers
  in acute coronary syndromes,
    17, 19
  in atrial fibrillation, 79
  in dilated cardiomyopathy, 31
  in hypertension, 91
  in stable angina, 15
Bicuspid aortic valve, 62–63
Blood pressure
  in aortic dissection, 96
  in cardiogenic shock, 35
  in cerebrovascular accident, 107
  in hypertension, 90–92
  in hypertensive emergency, 94
  in stable angina, 15
Bradycardia, in syncope, 9
Brain natriuretic peptide
  in dilated cardiomyopathy, 30
  in dyspnea, 5
  in systolic heart failure, 22
Buerger's disease, 111

C

Calcium channel blockers
  in atrial fibrillation, 79
  in hypertension, 91
  in Prinzmetal's (variant) angina, 13
  in stable angina, 15

Cannon "a" waves
  in atrioventricular nodal reentrant
    tachycardia, 86
  in second-degree heart block, 72
  in third-degree heart block, 74
  in ventricular tachycardia, 88
  in wide complex tachycardia, 76
Cardiac arrest, 10–11
Cardiac catheterization
  in aortic insufficiency, 53
  in aortic stenosis, 49
  in atrial septal defect, 61
  in cardiac arrest, 11
  in cardiogenic shock, 35
  in constrictive pericarditis, 43
  in mitral regurgitation, 51
  in mitral stenosis, 47
  in myocardial infarction, 19
  in pericardial tamponade, 41
  in pulmonary hypertension, 109
  in pulmonary stenosis, 65
  in right heart failure, 27
  in tricuspid regurgitation, 55
  in ventricular septal defects, 59
  in ventricular tachycardia, 89
Cardiac contusion, 114–115
Cardiac enzymes
  in cardiac arrest, 11
  in cardiac contusion, 114
  in myocardial infarction, 16, 18
  in myocarditis, 32
  in Prizmetal's (variant) angina, 12
  in ventricular tachycardia, 89
Cardiogenic shock, 34–35
Cardiomyopathy
  dilated, 30–31
  hypertrophic, 28–29
Cardioversion
  in atrial fibrillation, 79
  in atrial flutter, 81
Cardioverter-defibrillator
  in dilated cardiomyopathy, 31
  in hypertrophic cardiomyopathy, 29
  in sudden cardiac death, 11
Carotid bruit, 102–103
Carotid endarterectomy, 103
Carotid sinus massage
  in atrioventricular nodal reentrant
    tachycardia, 87
  in sick sinus syndrome, 82

  in syncope, 8
  in wide complex tachycardia, 77
Carvedilol, in systolic heart failure, 23
Cerebrovascular accident, 106–107
Chest pain, 2–3, 14–15, 16–17, 44
Chest radiography
  in adult congenital heart disease, 69
  in aortic coarctation, 100
  in aortic dissection, 96
  in aortic insufficiency, 53
  in aortic stenosis, 48
  in atrial septal defect, 60
  in bicuspid aortic valve, 63
  in cardiac contusion, 114
  in cardiogenic shock, 34
  in chest pain, 3
  in constrictive pericarditis, 42
  in diastolic heart failure, 24
  in dilated cardiomyopathy, 30
  in Dressler's syndrome, 45
  in dyspnea, 5
  in endocarditis, 56
  in hypertensive emergency, 94
  in mitral regurgitation, 50
  in mitral stenosis, 46
  in myocardial infarction, 18
  in pericardial effusion, 39
  in pericardial tamponade, 40
  in pulmonary hypertension, 108
  in pulmonary stenosis, 64
  in right heart failure, 26
  in systolic heart failure, 22
  in tricuspid regurgitation, 54
  in ventricular septal defects, 58
  in wide complex tachycardia, 76
Cigarette smoking, thromboangiitis
    obliterans and, 110
Cilostazol, in peripheral arterial disease, 99
Clopidogrel, in myocardial infarction, 17
Clubbing, 56
Cobalamin, in hyperhomocystinemia, 121
Cocaine abuse, 12
Colchicine, in Dressler's syndrome, 45
Commotio cordis, 114
Computed tomography
  in aortic coarctation, 101
  in aortic dissection, 97
  in cerebrovascular accident, 107
  in constrictive pericarditis, 43
  in hypertensive emergency, 95

in Marfan syndrome, 67
in secondary hypertension, 93
in transient ischemic attack, 105
Congenital heart disease, adult, 68–69
Congestive heart failure, 10
Contusion, cardiac, 114–115
Coronary calcium score, 122–123
Corrigan's pulse, 52
C-reactive protein, 118–119
Creatine kinase
    in cardiac contusion, 114
    in myocardial infarction, 16
    in myocarditis, 32
Cushing's reflex, 94, 106
Cushing's syndrome, 93

D
De Musset's sign, 52
Diastolic heart failure, 24–25
Diet
    in diastolic heart failure, 25
    in dilated cardiomyopathy, 31
    in hyperhomocystinemia, 120–121
    in hyperlipidemia, 117
Digoxin
    in atrial fibrillation, 79
    in atrial flutter, 81
    in complete heart block, 75
    in dilated cardiomyopathy, 31
Diltiazem, in Wolff-Parkinson-White
    syndrome, 85
Diuretics
    in constrictive pericarditis, 43
    in dilated cardiomyopathy, 31
    in diastolic heart failure, 25
    in right heart failure, 27
    in systolic heart failure, 23
    in tricuspid regurgitation, 55
Dobutamine stress testing, 21
Dopamine, in complete heart block, 75
Down's syndrome, 68
Dressler's syndrome, 44–45
Duroziez's sign, 52
Dyspnea, 4–5
    angina and, 2

E
Echocardiogram
    in aortic coarctation, 101
    in aortic insufficiency, 53
    in aortic stenosis, 49

in atrial fibrillation, 79
in atrial flutter, 80
in atrial myxoma, 113
in atrial septal defect, 61
in bicuspid aortic valve, 63
in cardiac arrest, 11
in cardiac contusion, 115
in cerebrovascular accident, 107
in complete heart block, 75
in constrictive pericarditis, 43
in diastolic heart failure, 24
in dilated cardiomyopathy, 31
in Dressler's syndrome, 45
in endocarditis, 57
in first-degree heart block, 71
in hypertrophic cardiomyopathy,
    28–29
in left ventricular hypertrophy, 125
in Marfan syndrome, 67
in mitral regurgitation, 51
in mitral stenosis, 47
in myocarditis, 33
in pericardial effusion, 39
in pericardial tamponade, 41
in pericarditis, 37
in pulmonary hypertension, 109
in pulmonary stenosis, 65
in right heart failure, 27
in sick sinus syndrome, 83
in stress testing, 21
in syncope, 9
in systolic heart failure, 22
in thromboangiitis obliterans, 111
transesophageal, 97
in transient ischemic attack, 105
transthoracic, 105, 107, 109
in tricuspid regurgitation, 55
in ventricular septal defects, 59
in ventricular tachycardia, 89
in wide complex tachycardia, 77
Effusion, pericardial, 38–39
Electrocardiogram
    in adult congenital heart disease, 69
    in aortic coarctation, 100
    in aortic dissection, 96
    in aortic insufficiency, 52
    in aortic stenosis, 48
    in atrial fibrillation, 78
    in atrial flutter, 80
    in atrial myxoma, 112

Electrocardiogram (*continued*)
  in atrial septal defect, 60
  in atrioventricular nodal reentrant
    tachycardia, 86
  in bicuspid aortic valve, 63
  in cardiac arrest, 10–11
  in cardiac contusion, 114
  in cardiogenic shock, 34
  in cerebrovascular accident, 106
  in chest pain, 3
  in constrictive pericarditis, 42
  in diastolic heart failure, 24
  in Dressler's syndrome, 44
  in dyspnea, 5
  in first-degree heart block, 70
  in hypertensive emergency, 94
  in hypertrophic cardiomyopathy, 28
  in left ventricular hypertrophy,
    124–125
  in mitral regurgitation, 50
  in mitral stenosis, 46
  in myocardial infarction, 16, 18–19
  in myocarditis, 32
  in palpitations, 7
  in pericardial effusion, 39
  in pericardial tamponade, 40
  in pericarditis, 36
  in peripheral arterial disease, 98
  in Prizmetal's (variant) angina, 12
  in pulmonary hypertension, 108
  in pulmonary stenosis, 64
  in right heart failure, 26
  in second-degree heart block, 72–73
  in sick sinus syndrome, 82
  in stable angina, 14
  in stress testing, 20–21
  in syncope, 9
  in systolic heart failure, 22
  in third-degree heart block, 74
  in tricuspid regurgitation, 54
  in ventricular septal defects, 58
  in ventricular tachycardia, 88
  in wide complex tachycardia, 76
  in Wolff-Parkinson-White syndrome, 84
Electrolytes
  in cardiac arrest, 11
  in myocardial infarction, 16
  in second-degree heart block, 72
  in ventricular tachycardia, 88
  in wide complex tachycardia, 76

Electrophysiologic studies, in palpitations, 7
Endocarditis, 56–57
Event recorder, 9
Ewart's sign, 38

F
Fenoldopam, in hypertensive
    emergency, 95
Fibrates, in hyperlipidemia, 117
Folate, in hyperhomocystinemia, 121

G
Gastroesophageal reflux disease, 2

H
Heart block
  complete, 74–75
  first-degree, 70–71
  second-degree, 72–73
  third-degree, 74–75
Heart failure
  diastolic, 24–25
  right, 26–27
  systolic, 22–23
Heart murmur. *See* Murmur
Heart rate, in stable angina, 15
Heart sounds
  in aortic insufficiency, 52
  in aortic stenosis, 48
  in cardiac contusion, 114
  in cardiogenic shock, 34
  in diastolic heart failure, 24
  in dilated cardiomyopathy, 30
  in hypertension, 90
  in hypertrophic cardiomyopathy, 28
  in left ventricular hypertrophy, 124
  in mitral regurgitation, 50
  in mitral stenosis, 46
  in myocardial infarction, 16
  in pulmonary hypertension, 108
  in right heart failure, 26
  in systolic heart failure, 22
  in tricuspid regurgitation, 54
Heart transplantation, in
    myocarditis, 33
Hollenhorst plaques, 104
Holter monitor, 9
Holt-Oram syndrome, 68
Homocysteine, 120–121
Hydralazine
  in dilated cardiomyopathy, 31
  in hypertensive emergency, 95

Hyperaldosteronism, 93
Hyperhomocystinemia, 120–121
Hyperlipidemia, 116–117
Hypertension
    aortic coarctation and, 100–101
    aortic dissection and, 2
    diastolic heart failure and, 25
    essential, 90–91
    in left ventricular hypertrophy, 125
    pulmonary, 108–109
    secondary, 92–93
Hypertensive emergency, 94–95
Hypertrophic cardiomyopathy, 28–29
Hypothermic therapy, in cardiac arrest, 11

I
Iloprost, in thromboangiitis obliterans, 111
Infection, endocardial, 56–57
Ischemic cerebrovascular accident, 106–107

J
Janeway lesions, 56
Jugular venous pressure, in pericardial
        tamponade, 40
    in constrictive pericarditis, 42
    in right heart failure, 26
    in systolic heart failure, 22
    in tricuspid regurgitation, 54

K
Kussmaul's sign, 40, 42

L
Labetalol, in hypertensive emergency, 95
Left ventricular hypertrophy, 124–125
Lipid panel
    coronary calcium score and, 123
    in C-reactive protein elevation, 118
    in hyperhomocystinemia, 120–121
    in hyperlipidemia, 116
    in stable angina, 15
Livedo reticularis, 34
Lungs, examination of, 4

M
Magnetic resonance angiography, in
        carotid bruit, 103
Magnetic resonance imaging
    in aortic dissection, 97
    in atrial myxoma, 113
    in constrictive pericarditis, 43
    in hypertensive emergency, 95

    in Marfan syndrome, 67
    in secondary hypertension, 93
    in transient ischemic attack, 105
Marfan syndrome, 66–67
MASS syndrome, 67
Medication history
    in cardiac arrest, 10
    in heart block 70, 72, 74
    in palpitations, 6
    in stress testing, 20
    in syncope, 8
    in wide complex tachycardia, 76
Metoprolol, in myocardial infarction,
        17, 19
Mitral regurgitation, 50–51
Mitral stenosis, 46–47
Muller's sign, 52
Murmur
    in adult congenital heart disease, 68
    in aortic insufficiency, 52
    in aortic stenosis, 48
    in atrial myxoma, 112
    in atrial septal defect, 60
    in bicuspid aortic valve, 62
    in cardiogenic shock, 34
    in endocarditis, 56
    in hypertrophic cardiomyopathy, 28
    in mitral regurgitation, 50
    in mitral stenosis, 46
    in tricuspid regurgitation, 54
    in ventricular septal defects, 58
Myocardial infarction
    non-ST segment elevation, 16–17
    ST elevation, 18–19
    tamponade and, 41
Myocarditis, 32–33
Myxoma, atrial, 112–113

N
Neurocardiogenic syncope, 8–9
Neurologic examination
    in cardiac arrest, 11
    in carotid bruit, 102
Nicardipine, in hypertensive emergency, 95
Nitrates
    in dilated cardiomyopathy, 31
    in stable angina, 15
Nitroglycerin
    in hypertensive emergency, 95
    in myocardial infarction, 17
    in Prinzmetal's (variant) angina, 13

Non-steroidal anti-inflammatory drugs
    in Dressler's syndrome, 45
    in pericarditis, 37
Noonan's syndrome, 64–65
Nuclear scanning, in stress testing, 21

O
Oliguria, 34
Osler's nodes, 56

P
Pacemaker
    in complete heart block, 75
    in sick sinus syndrome, 83
Pain
    chest, 2–3, 14–15, 16–17, 44
    pericardial, 36
    pleuritic, 2, 36
Palpitations, 6–7
Percutaneous catheter ablation, in atrial
    flutter, 81
Percutaneous coronary intervention, in
    cardiogenic shock, 35
    in ST elevation myocardial infarction, 19
Pericardial effusion, 38–39
Pericardial knock, 42
Pericardial rub, 38
Pericardial stripping, 43
Pericardial tamponade, 40–41
Pericardiocentesis, 37, 39, 41
Pericarditis, 33
    acute, 36–37
    constrictive, 42–43
    post-MI (Dressler's syndrome), 44–45
Peripheral arterial disease, 98–99
Persantine stress testing, 21
Phentolamine, in hypertensive
    emergency, 95
Pheochromocytoma, 93
Post-pericardiotomy syndrome, 45
Prinzmetal's (variant) angina, 12–13
Pulmonary embolism, 4
Pulmonary hypertension, 108–109
Pulmonary stenosis, 64–65
Pulse
    in aortic dissection, 96
    in atrial fibrillation, 78
Pulse volume recording, 99
Pulsus paradoxus, 40
Pulsus parvus et tardus, 62
Pyridoxine, in hyperhomocystinemia, 121

Q
Quincke's sign, 52

R
Raynaud's phenomena, 110
Rheumatic fever, 47
Roth spots, 56

S
Septal ablation, in hypertrophic
    cardiomyopathy, 29
Shock, cardiogenic, 34–35
Sick sinus syndrome, 82–83
Sodium nitroprusside, in hypertensive
    emergency, 95
Splinter hemorrhages, 56
ST segment
    in cardiac arrest, 11
    in cardiogenic shock, 34
    in myocardial infarction, 16,
        18–19
    during stress testing, 21
Statins
    in aortic stenosis, 49
    in C-reactive protein elevation, 119
    in hyperlipidemia, 117
    after myocardial infarction, 17, 19
    in peripheral arterial disease, 99
Stenosis
    aortic, 48–49
    mitral, 46–47
    pulmonary, 64–65
Stress testing, 20–21
    in first-degree heart block, 71
    in hypertrophic cardiomyopathy, 29
    in stable angina, 15
    in ventricular tachycardia, 89
Sudden cardiac death, 10–11
Supraventricular tachycardia, 8
Syncope, 8–9
Systolic heart failure, 22–23

T
Tachycardia
    atrioventricular nodal reentrant,
        86–87
    supraventricular, 8
    ventricular, 88–89
    wide complex, 76–77
    in Wolff-Parkinson-White syndrome,
        84–85

Tamponade, pericardial, 40–41
Tetralogy of Fallot, 65
Thromboangiitis obliterans, 110–111
Thrombolytic therapy, in cerebrovascular
    accident, 107
    in ST elevation myocardial infarction, 19
Thumb sign, 66
TIMI score, 17
Transesophageal echocardiogram, in aortic
    dissection, 97
    in atrial fibrillation, 79
Transient ischemic attack, 104–105
Traube's sign, 52
Tricuspid regurgitation, 54–55
Troponin
    in cardiac contusion, 114
    in myocardial infarction, 16
    in myocarditis, 32
Tuberculosis, 37
Turner's syndrome, 68

V

Vagal maneuvers
    in atrioventricular nodal reentrant
    tachycardia, 87

    in wide complex tachycardia, 77
    in Wolff-Parkinson-White syndrome, 85
Valve replacement
    in aortic insufficiency, 53
    in aortic stenosis, 49
    in bicuspid aortic valve, 63
    in mitral regurgitation, 51
    in mitral stenosis, 47
Vasodilators
    in Prinzmetal's (variant) angina, 13
    in pulmonary hypertension, 109
Ventricular septal defects, 58–59
Ventricular tachycardia, 88–89
Vitamin B6, in hyperhomocystinemia, 121
Vitamin B12, in hyperhomocystinemia, 121

W

Water hammer pulse, 52
Wide complex tachycardia, 76–77
Williams syndrome, 64, 65, 68
Wolff-Parkinson-White syndrome, 84–85
Wrist sign, 66